D

Dr Mike Smith is ￼ lth
Medicine and Presic ng
Doctors. He was th ....er or the Family
Planning Association ₁₉₇₀–75 and their Honorary Medical
Adviser 1975–90. He is also a founder member of the
National Food Safety Advisory Centre Expert Panel.

He has been an expert guest on the *Jimmy Young
Programme* once a fortnight for 15 years; an expert guest on
LBC once a week for ten years; and the medical columnist/
editor on *Woman's Own* for 15 years. Between 1980 and 1984
he presented BBC1's health series *Looking Good, Feeling Fit*,
and from 1988–90 he was an expert guest on SKY TV's
Weekly Magazine. In April 1991 he was voted the TV and
Radio Doctors' 'Expert's Expert' in the *Observer* magazine's
series.

His other books include *Birth Control, How to Save Your
Child's Life, A New Dictionary of Symptoms* and *Dr Mike Smith's
Handbook of Over-The-Counter Medicines*.

Also in *Dr Mike Smith's Postbag* series:

Arthritis

Back-Pain

H.R.T.

DR MIKE SMITH'S

POSTBAG

STRESS

WITH MARGARET ROOKE

KYLE CATHIE LIMITED

First published 1993 by
Kyle Cathie Limited
3 Vincent Square
London SW1P 2LX

ISBN 1 85626 087 9

A CIP catalogue record for this title
is available from the British Library

Typeset by DP Photosetting, Aylesbury, Bucks
Printed and bound in Great Britain
by Butler & Tanner Ltd, Frome and London

CONTENTS

INTRODUCTION

Stress affects all of us every day of our lives. Yet through my experience as a GP, through the calls I receive on the *Jimmy Young Programme*, through the letters that come to me from *Woman's Own* readers, time and time again I've reached the same conclusion – recognising we're stressed, working out why and doing something about it isn't easy for anyone.

It can be easy enough to acknowledge the physical symptoms that can come with stress. Maybe we'll find out our blood pressure's high or our heart beat's occasionally irregular or our head seems to have a permanent ache. Maybe we'll realise we've been a bit touchy lately or that we lack energy.

But it's much harder to confess to ourselves and to others that we feel stressed. To many 'stress' is seen as something of a dirty word, a sign of not being able to cope, of not being good enough or even of being neurotic. Unlike catching flu or breaking a leg or some other clearly physical ailment, it doesn't seem a good, solid cause for concern – no one ever got a sick note from their parents excusing them from games at school because they were suffering from stress.

However, if we don't realise that we're over-stressed, we can't find a way to make life less stressful for ourselves. Our health suffers, our relationships suffer and we get less enjoyment and pleasure out of life.

I remember learning this the hard way when I first started broadcasting. There I was on national radio, talking to millions of people about back pain and shingles, and I remember my mind focusing away from what I was saying and on to my audience. With a jolt I realised I could be talking to the country's leading authority on the subject in question, who could be sitting at home scowling at what I was saying because I hadn't read his special paper published in the latest medical journal. The Queen could be out there among the millions listening, or the Prime Minister, or others with superb, expert advisers. Maybe they too would be picking holes in the advice I was suggesting.

A few weeks later I realised how stressed I was feeling about my radio appearances. By giving myself time to think things through and work out where I could go wrong, I learnt to cope much better with my pre-programme nerves. I concentrated not on the grand and the great and the multitude listening in, but on one vulnerable person who doesn't have access to specialists and who is sitting at home, maybe in pain, needing some of the information I was giving out.

Even then at times of increased tension I went back to my old ways. If, say, I had to read out a list of medicines which should or shouldn't be taken for a particular condition and realised seconds before I opened my mouth to speak that I'd mislaid it, images of millions of listeners hearing my blunder would fill my mind. Again I had to work out a way to survive and to react better to moments like that one. The method I developed was to be completely honest – to say, 'I'm sorry, I've lost that list of names but I'll have it for you shortly.' The audience wouldn't thank me for giving them false information, after all, and hopefully they would appreciate that anyone can mislay something.

Working on radio sounds like a glamorous way to make a living and obviously the thought that so many people are listening to you and that any slip-up will be relayed to each and every one of them can be very stressful. But high levels of stress aren't limited to the harassed broadcaster or to other high-profile professionals, like the brain surgeon in the operating theatre or the businessman in the hostile boardroom. If we have a partner, a friend, a lover, a parent, a child, a boss, an employee, we will have stress in our lives. Even if we don't have any of these, we will still suffer stress – loneliness and poverty are both big stressors.

Often we see stress as something negative – that can be the way it's portrayed and it's a trap I sometimes fall into myself. But stress isn't always a bad thing. In fact we *need* to experience it in our daily lives. Positive stress – or pressure – is necessary for us to operate well and to make the most out of life. When we have to rise to an occasion that demands a special performance we need that rush of adrenalin. It stimulates us and motivates us. It's often when we feel those butterflies fluttering in the tummy that we do the best we can. When stresses stop, life can feel flat, empty and boring. The adrenalin no longer flows, our energy level drops and depression and lethargy become much more likely.

Problems arise, however, if we are faced with more pressure than our minds and our bodies can cope with. The amount of stress we can handle varies hugely from person to person. One might feel stressed at the slightest hint of responsibility, or worry about a trivial remark they had overheard (especially if their self-esteem is low and bound up with what others think of them). They might feel very fragile emotionally and crumple after only a small change to their lifestyle. Another will be able to cope with a great many different events and remain in control, calm and logical.

So a challenge to one person might be stress to another and breaking point for a third. Your personality and your bodily make-up determine how much stress you can take before your reactions become abnormal or unhealthy, perhaps before those butterflies in the tummy become a constant flow of acidic gastric juices that burn a peptic ulcer in the stomach's lining, or before bed stops being a place for relaxation, fun and slumber and starts being a battle ground where you fight to get to sleep.

When we are over-stressed our bodies suffer because of their automatic stress response. This is a reaction we humans have to real or imagined challenges and dangers. When we're under pressure our bodies release adrenalin and noradrenaline and many similar substances called chatechol amines. These, together with other hormones, allow us to face up to worrying situations. Immediately the blood circulates quickly around the body, carrying the maximum amount of oxygen to our muscles. Our blood sugar rises which means extra energy is available so we are ready for action. A certain amount of these bodily stresses, and so a certain amount of stress, is good for performance. Too much and problems result.

It's easy to see stress looming when we're driving up to a seemingly endless traffic jam or when we've chosen the slowest moving supermarket queue and we're already late for an appointment. But stress isn't caused by either of these situations, neither is it caused by a tough job or a crying child or a disagreement with your partner. We feel stressed because of the way we react to these situations. It's easy to apportion blame elsewhere – to your boss for not giving you a rise, to your partner for forgetting your birthday, to your child for the state of her room – but the answer, when looking at how to bring down high levels of stress, may well be not to change your job or your partner, or bully your child into tidiness, but to change the way you deal with them and react to them.

After all, if you decide you can't cope with your stressful existence and emigrate to Australia, you could well find yourself repeating the same patterns but on the other side of the world and with new companions. The scenery may be different, the stress will almost certainly be the same.

Similarly, if you leave a relationship because of all the stress you blame on your partner and your lives together, you may well find yourself with the same patterns of behaviour and similar stresses in the new bonds you form and in other parts of your life. What can seem like the answer may not be. The answer lies with you and the way you relate to problems and difficulties. And that can be harder to change.

Blaming others or other things is a big hobby of the stressed. Stress can often result from problems in our relationships, but if our relationship with ourselves has gone awry then we tend to offload more and more on to our nearest and dearest. Our stress cycle continues – and we are at the very heart of our own stress cycle.

So that's one common misconception about our stress levels – that they're someone else's fault. Another is that suffering from high levels of stress is a twentieth-century disease. In this century, in the wealthy West, we don't face many of the stressful conditions of yesteryear. In some parts of the world people are still coping with not knowing if there's enough food to get them through the week, but in this country most of us don't live with day-to-day cold and hunger. We can control our fertility, we can take holidays and we don't have to work the sort of slave-driving hours which used to be commonplace.

However, the modern lifestyle does bring particular pressures, particular physical and mental problems. These can be financial, or to do with work, or be related to the way families nowadays tend not to be based in small communities. There's also a stress which comes from watching terrible tragedies and scenes of violence on the television and being powerless to intervene to a large degree.

The company executive is the stereotypical twentieth-century stress victim. He's seen – and it's often the reality – as being under constant pressure to do better and better (although the pressure is often from himself). He has a car phone and a car fax and a bleeper, so he's rarely completely off duty. Especially in a time of recession he does have a stressful lifestyle, but repetitive jobs can be just as stressful. So can the loneliness of the mother at home with children and no adult company.

As I've already mentioned, I've noticed during my years as a doctor that quite often those people suffering most from stress tense up at the suggestion of it and deride the very thought of it. They see anything to do with relaxation as by its very nature unimportant and less of a priority than the really vital tasks of making money or getting the children to eat every scrap on their plates.

Yet we all need to have time for ourselves. We need to love and be loved, to have nourishing food, sleep, pleasant exercise and work that fulfils us, either at home or in a paid job. We also need to feel at peace with ourselves, to feel balanced and healthy. These are our emotional, physical and spiritual requirements. When our needs are out of balance, when overwork causes us to neglect ourselves or our families, again we can suffer from the effects of too much stress, which can lead to peptic ulcers, colitis, asthma, high blood pressure, migraine, coronary heart disease or many other stress-related illnesses. It can also lead to us being generally less pleasant and less stimulating to be with.

Some people, unable to cope with stress by giving proper attention to their needs, turn to drugs or alcohol as a means of relief. Unfortunately these are not only stressful substances for the body to cope with, but in turn can lead to dependence, addiction and illness – and undoubtedly to extra stress for partners, relatives or friends.

So this book has a bit of an up-hill task. It aims to indicate when stress might be having a bad effect on your mind and body, and to show healthier ways of tackling stress-related problems than ignoring them or trying to drown them in alcohol or shroud them in a haze of tobacco smoke.

When I sat down to think about the people who might be interviewed for this book it didn't take me long to think of an excellent case history very close to home. My own! In the past I've sometimes felt almost addicted to my own adrenalin, especially the adrenalin created when I'm working and pleased with my achievements. I've had to establish that I need to tackle the problem of my own stress. I've done this by making sure I create regular time for myself in which I can regain the emotional and physical balance I've already described. As you may have guessed, I am by nature a workaholic – I'm sure my wife would testify to that – and through the years I've established that giving myself time to regain this balance actually helps me work more effectively.

If I take some exercise regularly, spend time with my family, my pets, my garden and myself, if I listen to some music, give myself permission simply to sit and think and relax, my efficiency and energy improve manyfold. Maybe this is the best way to sell relaxation to a workaholic – it really does help you work more effectively.

We do need to focus on ourselves. There are ways we can help ourselves and accept help from others, and that is what this book is about. If you avoid facing up to the excess stress in your life, the consequences will come back to haunt you. If you face up to too much stress, if you notice it and acknowledge it, you are on your way to a less stressful, more balanced life – and a healthier, happier one too.

THE STRESSFUL SITUATION

SYMPTOMS

When we have too much stress in our lives we can be storing up all sorts of problems for ourselves. The reason for this is quite straightforward – the way we live in modern times has meant our bodily response to stress is many centuries out of date.

As I've already said, the body has an automatic response to anything which might be either frightening or pleasurable. It produces the hormones adrenalin and noradrenaline which flow into the blood stream, causing the heart rate to go up and sugars and fats to be released into the blood, providing instant energy.

In caveman times the hormones were used up by the necessary response to whatever was causing the stress. The troubled caveman either stayed to fight the creature or adversary that was threatening him or he turned on his heels and fled. But in most of today's stressful situations we can't just run away or physically battle it out. This means the adrenalin in the body which is still prepared, ready to be used in fight or flight, is bottled up instead. We no longer need the amounts produced inside our bodies and this is what eventually causes harmful stress.

So, although you may not be aware of it, if your circumstances at work or at home are constantly stressful or unhappy your body will be continually producing unneeded adrenalin. The various physical and emotional symptoms I've already described can then occur as well as many others which can range from indigestion to diarrhoea to a lack of sexual desire and very many others . . .

A Shopping List of Stress Symptoms

- Changes in sleep patterns including insomnia, early morning waking or alternatively excessive sleepiness and over-sleeping.
- Fatigue – lethargy in the mornings is a common example.
- Digestion changes – nausea, stomach aches, diarrhoea and, in extreme cases, vomiting.
- Appetite changes – eating too little or too much.
- Eating disorders, such as compulsive eating of binge foods, anorexia, bulimia.
- Drinking too much alcohol or taking illegal drugs to escape from feelings and to unwind.
- Smoking to calm yourself.
- Depression or feeling tearful, low, guilty or worthless.
- Bursts of temper or rage.
- Restlessness.
- Crying easily when it doesn't feel appropriate.
- Feelings of emptiness.
- 'Letting yourself go' – paying little attention to clothes, good food, your home and generally looking after yourself.
- Constantly thinking of past events, pains and what people said to you.
- Impatience and irritability.
- Fidgeting, clasping your hands or holding your arms across your body.
- Nail-biting.
- Difficulty in making decisions.
- Lack of concentration – losing track of conversations.
- Memory lapses.
- Lack of sexual drive and interest, or greatly increased sexual drive and interest to an uncomfortable level.
- Headaches.
- Aches and pains in other parts of the body – back and chest pains are common.
- Infections.
- Indigestion.

- Dizziness, faintness and fainting, sweating, twitching and trembling.
- Tingling of hands and feet.
- Breathlessness – breathing too fast and too deeply.
- 'Jelly' knees.
- Spots before the eyes.
- Palpitations – feeling very rapid heartbeats.
- Missed heartbeats – a sense of the heart standing still, then thumping.
- Panic attacks – waves of fear with sweating, trembling and a sense of impending death.
- Hypochondria – constant fear of physical illness, such as cancer, and identification of apparent symptoms.
- Feeling critical and uninterested in people.
- Finding it difficult to show your emotions from anger to joy.
- Feeling no one's looking after you.
- Shying away from being touched and from touching yourself and other people.
- Obsessive actions – cleaning, washing, counting or checking.
- Noises in the head.
- Slowness of speech.
- Hot and/or cold flushes.
- Facial flushing and pallor.
- Choking sensations.
- Lump or tightness in the throat.
- Dry mouth, difficulty in swallowing.
- Hair loss.
- Frequency in passing water.

These are some of the possible immediate stress symptoms, making it clear that well-being will suffer if care isn't taken. Illnesses with a clear link to stress include:

Asthma. This is an allergic reaction to various 'triggers' in which breathing becomes difficult. We take air in and out of the lungs through the bronchial tubes which secrete a small amount of mucus. During an attack there is an over-production of mucus, which narrows the tubes and thus makes breathing harder. In addition, the tubes get narrower, also as a result of the inflammation of their lining. Many different stressors can cause an attack, even a heavy meal which may have a stressful effect on the body.

Peptic Ulcer. A mucus is secreted from the lining of the stomach to protect it from the acids used in the breaking down of food and from other irritants. An ulcer occurs if there is a gap in this mucus protection and the acid attacks the stomach lining, or the oesophagus (the tube which leads to the stomach) or the small intestine. Going long hours without food makes ulcers more likely as food helps to neutralise the acid.

Irritable Bowel Syndrome. This has various symptoms including constipation and diarrhoea, sometimes intermittently, lower back pain, heartburn and fluid retention.

Hypertension. This means abnormally high blood pressure. In spite of what is often said, stress is rarely the cause of the kind of high blood pressure that persists and needs to be treated with medicines. But when we are under stress and get ourselves worked up and into a state, our blood pressure will usually rise, temporarily, until we settle down.

Eczema. This is also called dermatitis and involves inflammation of patches of the skin, often inside the knees and elbows or alternatively on the scalp and eyebrows.

Some experts believe controlling stress is also an important factor in beating cancer and rheumatoid arthritis and that the state of the emotions is vital in the prevention or development of these diseases. However, others disagree and say there's no evidence which shows that cancer, for example, can be stopped with psychological change. I believe that with cancer, the personality and attitude of the sufferer can play a large part in hampering the progression of the disease. Research has shown that those who are determined to fight it, as well as those who 'put it out of their mind', lead longer and better lives on average than those who just seem to 'give up'.

We're most likely to get ill in our weakest place. If we have a 'weak' throat it's likely that's where our stress will affect us, maybe with a tightness there. If our digestion causes us problems maybe we'll find ourselves with severe indigestion at stressful times. If our skin or eyes are a weak link, we may find a sudden smattering of spots or an eye infection hits us. And if you think someone is a pain in the neck that may actually be what they end up giving you . . .

Body Language

If it's not always easy to recognise when we're over-stressed, our body language might give us some clues. Unconscious tension is stored in the body and inevitably this will show itself. Maybe it's easier to spot in others and for others to spot in us. We've all seen people smiling away while they talk about a great time they've had while at the same time their bodies are telling another story. Maybe their jaw is rigidly clenched or their shoulders hunched up so much that you can't see their neck. They may be sitting with legs tightly crossed and their feet held upright and tense, as if wanting to be ready to run but also scared to leave. Their eyes might be darting about desperately avoiding eye contact or fixed to a particular spot on the floor, again avoiding your gaze. It's an idea to check on your own posture and eye movements and what they might be saying about the amount of tension within your own body.

STRESSFUL SITUATIONS

If you do recognise these symptoms in your body or your behaviour the next step could be to work out what it is you're reacting to to cause these stresses. The situation may be obvious or it may be less clear and you may need to give yourself some time to work through what might have triggered your symptoms. This isn't always straightforward. Confusingly, a very happy and exciting experience – getting married, a new baby, a big party, a new love affair – can be very stressful. If you've been through any sort of major life change it might be easier to spot this as the cause of your stress than if it is due to a lack of life changes and to you being in a bit of a rut.

Quite often too much stress can be obvious to everyone except the sufferer, so it's worth listening to the feedback of others – although, conversely, if you are over-stressed they will probably be trying to communicate with you at your most impatient.

Some causes of stress are pretty universal. In these uncertain economic times the mental health charity Mind suggests that fear of redundancy, of the recession and performance at work are overtaking personal problems such as bereavement, divorce and moving house as the main causes of stress.

Traditionally it's human relationships which are thought to be the main source of stress: J. Macdonald Wallace, a Health Education consultant on stress, sees the relationship between spouses as the main source, closely followed by the relationship between parent and child. The theory is that the home, as well as being the centre of affection and love, is also the location where we are most likely to be verbally, emotionally or physically battered.

Stress at Home

Where there are two people operating closely together there will naturally be conflicting views and ideas and, as has already been mentioned, it's how we react to these which is the key. When there are the added stresses of motherhood and fatherhood life becomes still more complicated and conflicts become more likely. Parenthood is a very stressful occupation. There's deadline after deadline, with no pay, no sickness benefits and no holidays – although there are, of course, other benefits! I remember the stresses my wife

Iona faced when we brought our first child back from hospital. The disturbed nights, and the nappies! We seemed to be surrounded by piles of them – washed ones, drying ones and in those days there were no washing machines and driers to help.

A few years on, the stress for Iona increased when I had to live in at the hospital in London during various stages of my medical training and was only home one and a half weekends a month and an occasional day in the week if I was lucky! I remember us discussing the loneliness she felt at not having adult company and the anxiety of being alone at night. This must affect a lot of women whose husbands travel, especially with the amount of movement there is with jobs at the moment.

Those with the biggest stress problem are thought to be working mothers. In a recent survey, 94 per cent of women with a job and children under sixteen said they suffered from stress. They felt their hardest task was finding time to get everything done, to sort their work problems, to look after the children and to cope with all their own daily pressures. Women receive mixed messages from society, about 'being a good mother and staying at home with the children' and about 'being an independent woman, going out to work and having it all'. What's also certain is that 'new men' aren't everywhere – in a typical home the mother is more likely to be doing the bigger share of housework and childcare than the father. If both partners are working, her share of worry and responsibility is therefore bigger.

Another pattern is for the father to take on the family's financial burden without sharing any of his concerns or fears with his partner, and for the mother to spend her time and energy listening to everyone else's problems but her own. Here, too, it's likely that arguments, disagreements, misunderstandings, resentments and depression, which could have been avoided, might come to the fore.

Very many stressful situations have their focus in the home and family, from illness and death of a loved one to divorce and financial worries. These 'home-based' stressors

figure strongly in the Holmes and Rahe Social Readjustment Rating Scale, which is the best known chart of change
and how much stress it can bring. Scores of around 300 in
a year are meant to indicate a major life crisis in some
individuals, scores of 200 to 299 a moderate life crisis and
100 to 199 a mild life crisis.

THE HOLMES AND RAHE SOCIAL READJUSTMENT RATING SCALE

Situation	Stress Factor
Death of a spouse	100
Divorce	73
Marital separation	65
Jail sentence	63
Death of a close family member	63
Personal injury or illness	53
Marriage/engagement/living together	50
Loss of job	47
Marital reconciliation	45
Retirement	45
Change in health of family member	44
Pregnancy	44
Sex difficulties	39
Birth of baby	39
Business readjustment	39
Change in financial state	38
Death of a close friend	37
Change to a different line of work	36
Change in numbers of rows with spouse	35
A large mortgage or loan	31
Foreclosure of mortgage or loan	30
Change in responsibilities at work (promotion or demotion)	29
Son or daughter leaving home	29
Trouble with in-laws	29
Outstanding personal achievement	28
Spouse begins or stops work	26

Beginning or end of school or college	26
Change in living conditions	25
Change in personal habits (more or less exercise)	24
Trouble with the boss	23
Change in work hours or conditions	20
Moving house	20
Change in school or college	20
Change in recreation	19
Change in church activities	19
Change in social activities	18
A moderate mortgage or loan	17
Change in sleeping habits	16
Change in rate of family gatherings	15
Change in eating habits, such as dieting	15
Holiday	13
Christmas	12
Minor violations of the law	11

While it's not possible to control some of the above, it is possible to control others and so keep your rating scale down for a twelve-month period. So, if you're changing jobs it might be best to leave moving house or taking out a huge bank loan until a later date.

But then, of course, we all react differently to all of the above. The messages we give ourselves about guilt and ambition and the need to impress others, for example, might force us through harsh experiences without examining what they're doing to us and the effects they're having. Then we suffer from unhealthy stress. If we listen to our needs, gain the reassurance we want and keep in perspective, everything life seems to be remorselessly throwing at us, we can cope so much better.

So if a child is moving away from home, we can tell ourselves we don't mind, that we always knew it would happen one day, and steel ourselves without examining what we really feel. Or we can examine what our concerns are – maybe fixing up a regular time for the son or daughter to keep in touch. We can check out our fears both for ourselves and for them and thus create, in the longer term, more peace of mind.

Stress at Work

Just as a lot of 'battering' in its broadest sense is located in the home, so the workplace can be another location – I'm especially thinking of verbal bullying. There can be a great deal of stress in relations between bosses and their employees, for both sides, and in relations between colleagues. Stress can revolve around frustrations if promotion isn't forthcoming, unrewarded efforts or rewarded laziness, shoddy work and many other areas of working life discussed below.

Figures about the cost to the economy of stress-related disorders vary but they average out at these staggering statistics – in one year three million working days and £7 billion are lost to industry through stress. Most of us dread suffering from a bad back and having time off work, but the reality is that more working days are lost through stress-related ailments than bad backs. Proof, if any were needed, that we should extend our concern for our health away from just the traditional areas.

I found it fascinating to read the jobs listed by insurance companies as the most stressful kinds of work.

1. *Miner.* Miners often put up with poor working conditions and the possibility of physical danger. They're also part of a shrinking industry.

2. *Airline pilot.* The levels of responsibility and concentrations for pilots are huge.

3. *Policeman or woman.* Again, the police face possible dangers and there can also be a level of unpopularity with sections of the public.

4. *Journalist.* The journalist faces constant deadlines and a

great deal of competition and pressure to perform. Here, too, can be a level of unpopularity with the public.

5. _Dentist._ Again, there's some unpopularity here – most of us don't leap about with joy at the thought of a dental check-up. Some dentists complain their work is tedious and uninteresting.

6. _Actor._ For most actors their working life is insecure and they often find themselves 'between jobs' or 'resting'. So there can be financial pressures, competition with others and the constant need to perform publicly to the best of their ability.

7. _Prison officer._ Another unpopular job. Prison officers often suffer from undermanning at work. They can fear attack from prisoners and can feel cooped up at their places of work.

8. _Doctor._ We doctors, the experts say, find life stressful because of the long hours and because of the level of responsibility we have for others in listening to complaints and troubles (and so soaking up the stress of others), diagnosing their conditions, prescribing a cure and carrying out surgery. Many in my profession are facing alcoholism or drug abuse, depression, suicide and marital breakdown, according to a report for the British Medical Association.

9. _Nurse._ Overworked and underpaid as everyone knows and objects to.

10. _Television and radio star._ I've mentioned earlier in this book, the pressures of live performance.

For a longer, less stressed life the following are recommended as ideal careers:

1. _Librarian._ The work of a librarian is generally seen as guaranteeing a tranquil life.

2. *Museum curator.* The museum curator often has pleasing work to attend to in a calm and cultured atmosphere.

3. *Vicar.* The local religious leader again has a calming atmosphere at work. He's likely to feel committed to his work and often receives appreciation from the community he serves.

4. *Beautician.* The beautician can see instant results from her work which is a very pleasing reward, as is an obvious improvement in the esteem and mood of her client. The work can be very relaxing and compliments and appreciation are likely.

5. *Occupational therapist.* This is rewarding work and the occupational therapist, too, is likely to hear appreciation from his or her patients.

6. *Bank clerk.* The bank clerk has a good understanding of money which is an area of life that can cause great stress to those of us who may not. He or she will also benefit from cheap mortgages. Unlike the policeman, journalist or prison officer, there's a physical boundary between the bank clerk and even the most unpleasant customer.

7. *Gardener.* Gardening is found by millions to be very therapeutic as a hobby and it can be too for those who make it their living.

8. *Dietician.* The dietician has an understanding of healthy eating and healthy lifestyles – crucial for keeping levels of stress healthy too.

9. *Insurance broker.* The insurance broker's work is seen as secure and well paid.

10. *Computer programmer.* The work of a computer programmer is seen as rewarding and as a job for the future as we see more and more computer equipment in our daily lives.

I'm sure some of you reading this second list are already

seething with indignation. The computer programmer with poor eyesight as a result of staring at the screen and the librarian struggling with cutbacks in library services are likely to feel misrepresented on the above list. In fact, just to show that there are always exceptions – and two sides to every argument – it was reported recently that a special country club has been established for members of the clergy to help them rest, relax, recharge their spiritual batteries and recover from the pressures of their work.

Research has shown that senior staff who have more control over their working lives find life less stressful than those who obey orders rather than giving them. So it's interesting that doctors are mentioned on the above list, but there's no sign of hospital orderlies and cleaners.

Others have also been left out of these lists which different research might suggest should have been there. The teaching profession, with its many recent changes in curriculum and exam structure, is one which faces a great deal of stress – more, according to a Birmingham University report, than those typically thought to be over-stressed, such as company directors and middle managers. It's also been reported that an advice bureau has been established for stressed farmers who've been hit by the recession, who feel their status has gone down over the years, whose lives are isolated, and who may feel that with economic difficulties they've let down the previous generations who successfully farmed their land.

Stress at work can be due to a wide range of issues, from periods of great activity – too much to do and too little time – to worries about redundancy. Whatever the catalyst, when we're over-stressed we are less efficient and more prone to accidents. The trend towards stress counselling in the workplace shows that despite the British stigma about emotional and mental problems and the supposed need to keep a stiff upper lip at all times, employers are beginning to realise that they're not employing part of the person part of the time, but the whole people whose life outside work will affect life within it. Stresses from home can't be left at the factory gate or the office door.

Unemployment brings its own stresses, and not just financial ones. The lack of identity, direction and structure to the day and the low self-esteem which often accompany joblessness can make life more stressful and make finding another job less likely.

Another very stressful state of affairs can be running your own business. According to a Sunderland Polytechnic survey, being self-employed can be satisfying but it can also have adverse effects on health. Those who are their own boss complained they never seemed to be able to put the problems of business behind them. There was no escape, especially if they operated from home. They also tended not to take time off if they felt ill because they thought they couldn't afford it. The insecurity of income and the reliance on others to pay bills added to the pressure they felt.

In Britain we work some of the longest hours in Europe. Many of us have stayed on at work because everyone else is still there and we would feel lazy or less committed if we got up and went, even though our work's done. One friend of mine, Robert, is convinced his unpopularity at one job was due to him getting his work done to a high standard and then leaving at the time specified on his contract, with his colleagues scowling at him from behind their desks. He believes his boss was not only scowling along with them but was also jealous of his self-confidence and willingness not to conform with the company tradition when it ate into his social life. As he says, in other countries working very long hours is seen as a sign of inefficiency. In this country it's seen as a sign of dedication and devotion.

Stress at work can have countless roots, many of which have easily spotted equivalents in the home or the school or any other environment. Academics Cooper and Marshall have outlined some. Stress, they say, can result from poor working conditions – even dangerous ones – from having too much work or too little time to do it in, from being unsure of your role, from being responsible for others, from being under- or over-promoted, from lacking job security and seeing your ambitions disappear, from poor relations with bosses, subordinates or colleagues to problems with delegating, from having little or no participation in decision making and from office politics. The trend towards more short-term contracts and fewer full-time jobs adds to stress levels still further.

The *New York Times* published the following method of helping to spot stress at work.

STRESS AT WORK: CAUSES AND REMEDIES

Add the number of points indicated for each of these working conditions which produces stress.

Three points each: CAUSES
Company has been taken over recently
Staff reductions/lay-offs in past year
Department/company had major reorganisation
Staff expect company to be sold or relocated
Employee benefits significantly cut recently
Mandatory overtime frequently required
Employees have little control over how they do their work
Consequences of making a mistake at work are severe
Workloads vary greatly
Most work is machine-paced or fast-paced
Staff must react quickly and accurately to change
Personal conflicts are commonplace

Two points each:
Few available opportunities for advancement
Red tape hinders getting things done
Inadequate staffing, money or technology
Pay is below the going rate
Sick and vacation benefits are below the norm
Employees are rotated between shifts
New machines/work methods have been introduced

Noise/vibration levels are high or temperature keeps changing

Employees normally isolated from one another

Performance of work units normally below average

One point each:
Employees have little or no privacy
Meal breaks are unpredictable
Work is either sedentary or physically exhausting

Add the number of points for these stress-reducing conditions.

Three points each: REMEDIES
Staff recognised and rewarded for their contributions
Management takes firm action to reduce stress
Mental health benefits are provided
Company has formal employee communications programme
Staff given information on coping with stress
Staff given clear job descriptions
Management and staff talk openly with one another
Employees are free to talk with one another

Two points each:
Work rules are published and the same for everyone
Child care programmes are available
Employees can work flexible hours
Perks are granted fairly
Employees have access to necessary technology
Staff and management trained in resolving conflicts
Staff receive training when assigned new tasks
Company encourages work and personal support groups
Staff have place and time for relaxation

One point each:
Staff assistance programme is available
Each employee's work space is not crowded
Staff can put up personal items in their work areas
Management appreciates humour in the workplace

Programmes for care of the elderly are available

Then subtract your total points for stress reducers from your total points for stress producers. The result may range from minus 50 points for excellent working conditions to plus 60 points for an extremely high stress environment.

HOW MUCH CAN WE TAKE?

However many points we and our place of work score, what this chart won't tell us is how much stress we can bear. Some of us are naturally more sensitive to stress than others, owing to inborn characteristics and experiences encountered during childhood and later.

A stable upbringing certainly helps counter the effects of stress and those who've had a traumatic childhood are more likely to suffer adversely. Too much stress will be what they grew up with and they come to regard it as the norm. So recognising it as something that's unhealthy will be much harder unless we're open to the opinions and perception of others. A difficult childhood is also likely to lead to low self-esteem, and so to over-dependence on others to provide a sense of emotional well-being and self-worth. But only *you* can give yourself that sense. Without it you may disbelieve or discount the praise and support of others. The hope that other people can fulfil all your needs will inevitably be dashed time and time again – a very stressful way to live. Dissatisfaction, frustration, anger, depression and hopelessness may result.

For women, the amount of stress they can handle before these symptoms erupt also depends on the time of the month. Pre-Menstrual Syndrome leaves many women feeling very tense and under the weather, and the time when women are ovulating can also affect the emotions. The state of an individual's health is another factor – when we're feeling good physically and psychologically it's easier to keep incidents in perspective.

The time of day can matter, too. If you're a morning person like me you'll know how astonishing it is to hear how angry and uptight others can get at not finding a matching pair of socks when they get up. Yet if I'm out with my wife and want to get home and find I'm stuck in a traffic jam or in a long conversation, that's when my blood's more likely to boil (though I have been known to fall asleep with the other person still talking. Not often, though. It's usually the other way around!).

The state of the relationships in your life will be another factor for your own personal stress scale.

The research that's been carried out into the personality types most likely to suffer from too much stress and stress-related conditions is quite fascinating. American heart experts Rosenman and Friedman carried out extensive research in the US and categorised the type of person most likely to have a heart attack. They grouped people into Type As and Type Bs and found that Type As, whose attitudes to life were more stressful, had seven times more coronary heart disease. So which are you?

Some of the characteristics of Type As are:

Bottling up feelings
Always competitive, plays to win
Always hurrying around and arriving everywhere
    early
Always watching the clock
Setting oneself deadlines
Hating being kept waiting, impatient
Often frowning, scowling and clenching fists
Thinking about other things while talking and listening
    with someone
Can't bear to be criticised
Hating to leave work unfinished
Trying to get others to get to the point when they're
    talking
Ask 'What am I achieving?' not 'Am I enjoying myself?'

Type Bs were more able to relax and play, were more laid back, could co-operate with other people more easily and could give themselves permission to ease off when they felt tired.

The 1980s could almost be called a Type-A decade, with its atmosphere of and emphasis on financial gain and competition. But even then bottling up feelings had its limits – during the decade, calls to the Samaritans almost doubled. The nineties have a different feel to them but both the recession and concerns about the environmental future of the planet have brought their own stresses that we must deal with.

It's easy to read in some of the Type-A characteristics listed above those of people who tend to be very critical and impatient of others' weaknesses and standards. I feel it's also important to notice how many on the list can also be directed towards ourselves. We can so easily be our own harshest critics. The clenched fist and scowl can be our reaction to something we've done or haven't done – a sign of our guilt or fierce ambition if we haven't reached the exacting, sometimes maybe impossible, standards we set ourselves.

The first on my list, 'bottling up one's feelings', is a very British trait and I do believe that if we don't examine our feelings, and keep our anger or our loneliness or our needs locked inside us, this will take its toll on our emotional well-being and even on our physical health.

But, of course, it's not always appropriate to show everyone how we're feeling all of the time. In some circumstances we must wear a fixed smile, and hold out a welcoming hand to shake when inside it's our whole body that's shaking. In a job interview, for example, bursting into tears due to nervousness probably won't impress. Likewise television newscasters have often described themselves as feeling like ducks in water: all that's on show is calm and unflappable and serene; underneath they're paddling like mad to stay afloat. I once heard one say that slipping up on a word or finding they were missing a vital piece of paper for the next story brought the same stress level as that of a minor road accident. Yet if any of this showed we viewers would be pretty astonished.

Perhaps both of these are examples of the way stress can be positive and negative. The negative side could be dealt with once the job interview or television broadcast is over – by exercising to use up some of the adrenalin that's been released, by relaxing and working through our feelings about what's just happened. The positive side helped us to thrive during the experience; rather than feeling bored and lethargic we were stimulated and full of energy and achieving our highest potential. We can deal more efficiently with a sudden frightening or difficult event which demands immediate action, and survive actions which, without the energy we gain from stress, would normally exhaust us. We can feel stimulated, excited, understanding, creative and lively. Without that energy we achieve less and feel inclined to achieve less.

WHEN THINGS GET BAD

If you have too little stress in your life negative feelings can take over. You'll still be searching for things to worry about even if you've hidden from big pressures and challenges, and you'll end up concentrating your fears on very small incidents, blowing them up out of proportion. Your energy levels will get lower and lower and you may well find the days and years go faster while you achieve much less in them.

But too much stress can commonly lead to anxiety and fear, which of course we can suffer to different degrees of intensity. A small amount of anxiety is called worry and this stays with us until the problem is sorted out. When a threat is more immediate and feels like a burden hanging over us, this is fear. An abnormal amount of this is called a phobia which is an intense fear of something which would not make the average person afraid, for example, confined spaces, spiders or flying in an aeroplane.

If any of these occur regularly it's easy to start to believe you have a serious illness because of the physical symptoms that anxiety and worry can bring on. Fear of this illness again fuels the stress as our mind and body give each other a vicious circle of messages. Sufferers may feel generally anxious and inadequate, perhaps at work or while socialising, even to the point of leaving their job and staying at home.

One particularly unpleasant symptom of stress is the panic attack. This is a shortlived period of intense fear with the belief that something terrible is about to happen. Adrenalin pours into the bloodstream, the heart thumps and the sufferer feels breathless or faint, has chest pains, and is convinced he or she is about to collapse – a very frightening experience. I've also heard sufferers say it's as if they're being choked or smothered and that generally they don't feel as if they're in the real world.

Andrew
The son of a family friend told me how he experienced a very frightening panic attack when his relationship with his girlfriend went wrong.

> Our relationship had never felt like plain sailing but I always thought we'd end up together. I'd told her I really wanted to get married and we set a date. But after that we didn't seem to be on the same wavelength at all. We were arguing much more. Linda couldn't make a positive decision about anything to do with the wedding. We had to try for ages to find a church which would marry us as I'd been married before. When we found one I was really pleased but Linda said she didn't like the church and it wasn't what she wanted so we had to keep looking.
>
> As the date grew nearer I started to panic slightly.

I'd say, 'We've got to get the invitations out, people are expecting this all to be organised.' But it was as if she couldn't hear me. I kept hanging on desperately to the thought that sooner rather than later we would find what she wanted and then everything would work out. My past experience of our relationship was that we didn't always communicate well but we loved each other and things would work out all right. I suppose I was thinking that, without looking too far ahead – without daring to.

Andrew says that looking back now he can see the relationship was doomed. At the time he was trying not to look at it at all.

Then one day, when there was only a couple of months to go and I thought things had improved a bit between us, she phoned. We were chatting about the wedding and the arrangements and I just knew there was something more she wanted to say. She didn't sound like herself at all. She wasn't drunk but I could tell she'd been drinking.

Then she said it. She said, 'I've got something else to tell you.' I felt sick as soon as she said those words. She started telling me she'd met this other man at a party and it had started her wondering whether she wanted to go through with the wedding. I was horrified. We'd been together so long I never dreamt, however bad our problems, that we wouldn't see them through together. It felt like she was part of my stability and my future and now both were being threatened and taken away from me.

Then all of a sudden she'd change tack and tell me she loved me and wanted to go through with it. Everything she said confused and frightened me more. Basically she didn't know what she wanted so I felt I had to draw it out of her. It was like a turkey voting for Christmas. There I was on the end of the phone persuading her to spell out all the doubts and misgivings she'd kept from me. Everything she said felt like torture – the wedding wasn't what she wanted.

I went to my bedroom feeling physically out of control. I felt hysterical but the tears weren't coming out. It was just all there inside me. I sat on my bed rocking backwards and forwards. I tried to speak but the words didn't come out. I think even then the implications of the conversation were so great I couldn't allow myself to think about everything that had been said. My mind would explode – along with my whole future.

It was a week later when it hit me. That's when I had the panic attack. It was one of the most unpleasant things I've ever felt – as if my mind and body were playing tricks on me. I was sitting on a train when suddenly it felt as if the train was turning round, as if I was no longer there but on some sort of fun-fair ride. I was actually leaning forward to try to stop being thrown out of my seat because I really felt as if that's what would happen. I felt very sick and very faint. The whole horrible experience kept pouring into my head. I couldn't escape it any more. It was the same feeling I'd had during the phone call which I hadn't allowed myself to feel since. Now I couldn't stop it.

The feeling was so big it felt as if it was crushing me – the knowledge that someone I'd believed would never let me down had done just that. I suffered for fifteen minutes, trying to stay upright while in my mind the train was moving round. I was sweating and sweating, trembling a bit too, I'm sure people were looking at me and not knowing what to do.

It felt as if all the things I couldn't bear to look at in my life all came and attacked me at once. It was a horrible experience. I'd never want that to happen again.

The panic attack is an extreme response to anxiety. The body's usual anxiety response – the outpouring of adrenalin, the increase in the heart beat and blood pressure and all the other signs – is a healthy one. Problems arise, however, when these reactions continue in normal circumstances. The response was not designed to cope with the pressures of continuous mental stress, which when bottled up can produce insomnia, tense and aching muscles, frightening feelings of panic, bouts of sweating and shaking, lack of concentration and irritability, and so many of the other symptoms I've already outlined. If this happens the system overloads and the immune and circulatory systems are damaged and our health suffers.

With anxiety and fear, symptoms can be triggered off by an event so insignificant we forget what it was. Fear then literally becomes blind terror – we cannot see what has led us to respond in the way we are. Those from anxious families may recognise how this is a part of their family life, when a day-to-day difficulty can have a huge effect and can lead to a full psychiatric illness such as a nervous breakdown.

There's also a relatively newly named phenomenon, Post-traumatic Stress Syndrome, which affects some people who've lived through a disaster such as an accident or a war. They may frequently experience the emotions they felt at the time of the trauma, possibly through nightmares, and may suffer distress in similar situations.

CHILDREN

I feel it's important to say something about stress and children partly because a lot of the ways we learn to cope with stress we learn when we are young. Many people are surprised when I say that children can suffer from stress –

it's easy to think, 'Adults have the responsibilities, so what can children have to worry about?' But there are many things – from arguing with a friend, to being left out of a 'gang', to losing a grandparent, to not being able to watch a favourite TV programme. A child has the same range of emotions as an adult even if he or she sometimes feels less able to communicate them. Children can feel resentful, put upon and responsible for situations – from a broken vase to their parents' divorce – yet are powerless to do anything to help the situation.

Sometimes children and adolescents express stress and anxiety as being bored, or like grown-ups they'll feel physical symptoms such as tummy aches and headaches. They'll have less ability to concentrate so their school work can suffer. Anxious children have a tendency to grow into anxious adults so it's very important that they be allowed to express their anxieties and are reassured and helped during stressful situations.

If there's a stressful event for you in your life, such as the birth of a new baby or a huge family gathering for Christmas, there are likely to be implications, too, for the stress levels of your child. At other times stressful situations are focused directly on the children, such as early romances or the lack of them, first days at new schools, or exams. One figure I've heard is that around 20,000 teenage girls a year take an overdose (apparently this affects girls more than boys) so it's vital not to underestimate the depth of your child's or your teenager's feelings and needs.

I've heard two stories recently which have confirmed this for me. One was a letter I received from a mother worried about her daughter who, she feels, is falling into the same trap as she did when she was young.

> I was more stressed when I was a teenager than at any other time. I always had too much to do, too much that had to be done. I set myself all sorts of goals all the time. I don't mean I had to get good exam results. I mean I wanted to be popular, thin,

have boyfriends, go out a lot in new clothes, all those sorts of things.

Somehow the teachers at school thought my priorities were different. They decided I was a coper and an organiser. I was the 'sensible one' and they heaped extra responsibilities on me. I was put on this committee and that committee. I enjoyed it in a way. It made me think, 'I'm popular, I'm wanted, I'm in demand.' I wanted to feel those things so I didn't say, 'No, I want to hang out with my friends.'

Now my daughter is the one on the school council organising the school dance just like I did and that worries me. When I was at school if I'd said, 'I don't want to be responsible for running the tuck shop,' I think the teachers would have said, 'Don't be ridiculous. We trust you to do it.' And I think the others would have said, 'Oh, go on, we won't have one unless you do it.' I felt as if I never really had any choice. I had to squeeze so much into my days. It felt like there was never any time for me, just to daydream and read magazines and look in the shops. I'd be running about in break time trying to make sure everyone was coming to this meeting who had said they would or that we could have such and such a room for a play rehearsal.

At the time I didn't know I was stressed. On top of the school extras and my school work I was doing what I wanted to do – going out with boys, going to parties. I remember being tired all the time.

I blamed my parents. I felt I'd have been all right if they hadn't made me wash the dishes. I just wanted to slump in a chair and watch *Coronation Street*. They had no idea I felt so exhausted and was so resentful. I'm sure they think, the teachers think, the other girls think, I sailed through it and loved doing it all. My daughter gives that impression too. She seems to love all the organisation and being at the centre of things. I just hope it's what she really wants to do.

Childhood is the time we develop many of our phobias, such as fear of heights, snakes, thunder or crowds. This is what happened to Janet, my second example, who developed a fear of exams.

At every exam it would be the same. Everyone else would be in there writing and writing for all they were worth. I'd just sit, shake and almost faint with the stress of the moment. Sometimes I'd actually burst out crying I was so terrified of being there and having to perform in the exam.

Every time my results were absolutely terrible. The school thought and my parents thought that I hadn't worked hard enough but what they didn't know was that I'd started to revise months early. My friends thought I was mad – I wouldn't go out with them, I'd stay at home and work instead. Every time I thought, 'If I work harder it will all be OK,' but every time it was tortuous.

Things came to a crisis for Janet in her third year – and that was when action and notice was taken.

It was a really easy Geography exam. I should have been able to do it with my eyes shut. All the others were laughing and joking outside the exam hall because it was a bit of light relief compared to the other tests we had. I started off all right which was pretty amazing for me but then I came to a question I couldn't answer. Instead of just going on to the next one I panicked. I started crying really loudly and shaking. I knew I was disturbing everyone so I got up and ran out of the classroom. I've never felt so embarrassed and stupid – and so disappointed in myself.

I wanted my parents to be proud of me and I wanted to be just like my friends – I didn't want to be brilliant, just average would have been fine. I felt I was letting them down, especially as they didn't understand.

No one did until a new form teacher spotted how much worse my exam results were than my work during the term. We sat down and had a really good talk about it which felt wonderful – just to be listened to felt such a relief. I took my next exams in a room all to myself which was much better for me and after a few I progressed to sitting at the front of the exam hall so I wasn't aware of lots of people scribbling away around me. Just a few practical measures and a sympathetic hearing made all the difference in the world to me.

SELF-HELP TREATMENT

As I've already suggested, with stress the first and most important step to finding a remedy is to recognise that you have a problem, when you have the problem and what you're able to do about it. Check how you're feeling and your physical and emotional symptoms against the list I gave in the previous chapter (see pages 9–12).

Especially if there is a lot going on in your life – or, on the other hand, if there is disappointingly little – give yourself some time to work out how stressed you are. Watch for the bodily signs – for example, the hunched shoulders which come when we feel threatened – or ask your partner or a friend if they've noticed any change in your posture or mood.

Start taking notice of triggers which bring out stress symptoms in you. What were you thinking, what was happening in your mind and body, what were you doing to bring on those reactions? Use the messages from your mind and body as a means to help you look after yourself.

TAKING CHARGE OF YOUR LIFE

To me there are few better ways of cutting down the amount of stress in your life than by taking a look at your lifestyle as if you were a fly on the wall. By examining your life from an objective position you may see options that don't feel possible when you're in the middle of your daily, hectic routine. If you have financial stresses, for example, maybe it will be clearer, from your objective position, to see where you can economise or change your spending patterns or how you can earn more money. If your job is mundane and unexciting maybe you can see how to argue for more responsibility or perhaps you can make the decision that this work isn't for you and you need to look for a change. If your home life and relationships are the focus of your discontent maybe you will be able to see ways to communicate this without attaching blame to the other people involved, or work out ways of making life happier and more satisfactory.

Sometimes from inside a difficult situation it feels impossible to make changes. Many times I've heard complaints from over-worked and over-stretched mothers of small children about how much they have to do and how little time they have to do it in. If the children are very active and very inquisitive or very dependent on their mother's company, she can feel she has no time for herself. It's hard to think of a more stressful situation than that.

This is just one example of a situation which can lead to extreme stress at home, and which can seem on one level to have no way out. The mother's needs aren't being met, her voice as an individual isn't being heard. It seems as if there's no time for her to do what she wants. If this sounds like you, see if there are some compromises that can be reached, if there's some housework you're doing as a matter of routine that really isn't essential, if there isn't some help you could get in looking after the children, even if just for a few hours. The routine can be changed and your priorities can be altered to include some time for you even if we're talking about a few minutes here and there while your child is in a play-pen or somewhere else safe and secure. If there aren't childminders and babysitters on hand, the possibility of an hour to yourself watching your favourite television programme or reading a good magazine may seem an impossible dream, but just *five minutes* spent thinking about yourself and how you are, while sipping a cup of tea and putting your feet up, can make all the difference.

Cutting down on whatever it is that stresses us isn't always a realistic proposition. For example, if you feel very stressed every time your baby cries, and you're doing everything you can to stop the tears, you will have to live with them. In that situation the ideal is to try to limit the damage to your nerves. If someone or something brings on a stress reaction in us it's because we see it or them as a threat to our well-being. So the message we might be hearing when our baby cries could be that we're no good as parents or that the baby's very ill. If we can find a way to comfort and talk to ourselves while we're feeling that stress, reminding ourselves of some of the good times as well as the bad, undoing some of the negative thoughts, we might find life slightly easier.

Writing lists of your priorities for the day is always a good way of organising yourself – and planning is a good way of beating stress. Just the mere fact that you're jotting down a list of your household chores gives you an opportunity to question what really needs to be done. I always think a good rule is that if a job isn't enjoyable and isn't worthwhile, don't do it. Delegating can be a very useful tool and don't underestimate the degree to which children can help – and may well enjoy helping. Another way of beating stress is to find some greenery. Walking in a park, sitting in your garden if you have one, or taking a small trip to the nearest bit of countryside can really take your mind off your problems and help get them into perspective. Even if it's cold or wet you can wrap up warm, grab an umbrella, and remind yourself that there's life outside the four walls of your home.

Other tips for cutting down the stress in your life include keeping things tidy. This is both safer, as there are fewer things to trip over, and also means you're less likely to lose something vital. And don't expect to be the best at everything – no one can be, and it can be uselessly stressful trying. Meeting deadlines by the skin of your chattering teeth is a sure way to make your blood pressure and headache rate rise, as is generally overloading yourself with things to do.

Make sure you get enough sleep but not too much. I have heard of people sleeping fifteen hours a day – for them staying in bed is comforting, it feels like a stress-free zone. But remember, depression often goes hand in hand with stress and people who are stressed aren't necessarily always on the go – that's a stereotype. Continual tiredness and a desire to sleep all day are among the main indicators of stress.

On the other hand, it may be that a part of you goes into overdrive and works until you're exhausted. That part feels this is more than fine – it's what's right and expected of you. If that's how you feel it's worth asking yourself where that message came from and why you follow it, rather than just accepting it as a fact of life. Maybe when you were a child that's what you were told to do – to work harder and harder rather than playing and enjoying yourself.

Through questioning whether the path we've always taken is the only possible one to tread, we may find a more balanced, healthy and fulfilling way of life. By standing one step away and looking at what we've got, we can set ourselves achievable targets to cut down on the routines and responsibilities that are keeping our stress levels high, and we can add to the part of our life that we associate with relaxation and fun.

Taking charge of your life means making sure all areas of your life have prominence and importance in your schedule. That may include some voluntary work – doing something you believe in – or finding a hobby that really excites you. It also means working out what you need to do to relax, perhaps having a bath, saying a prayer, sitting quietly or going for a swim. We're all different but we *all* need to give ourselves that time just for us.

Pauline

In my years as a doctor I don't think I have come across a group of people who face a more stressful existence day in and day out than 'carers', those who work full-time looking after a sick or disabled relative.

I feel Pauline's case is a very strong one. She is making the most out of a highly stressful and very difficult situation, keeping some time for herself which is fulfilling and brings her a sense of achievement.

She met her husband Les at a dancing school when she

was fifteen and he was twenty. They married several years later and had five daughters.

> We were very average, no different from any other family. With five daughters growing up there were plenty of stresses. There was always something to worry about as they became teenagers, grew into their twenties, got married and had families of their own.
>
> As they've now moved away from home I should be enjoying this time for myself. But I can't. I feel cheated. It's as if I'm looking after a child again. I have no freedom – I can't say, 'I'm going out,' or 'I'm going to be late.' I have this responsibility all the time.

The cause of Pauline's frustration is the stroke Les suffered five and a half years ago. Now he's fifty-five, but instead of looking forward to an active retirement with his wife, he's paralysed and dependent on her a great deal of the time. To Pauline he seems like a stranger. 'He's just like a child,' she explained. 'You can't have a proper conversation with him because he doesn't understand and he can't answer you back.'

Without warning, Les had two major strokes and lots of smaller ones. A year after his first he had another massive stroke.

> This left him unable to talk and unable to get out of bed. In hospital he had yet another stroke. I went to see him and he was jabbering away but when I got closer to him I realised he wasn't talking any sense. It felt like he was just this body in a bed. No one had phoned us to tell us he'd had another stroke and we thought he was just going to die.

Instead, the final stroke had left him paralysed down his

right-hand side, although since then there have been some improvements through physiotherapy.

'It was so hard to believe this was happening to me although I was living it,' says Pauline. After thinking he was going to die she swung round to believing he'd be back to full health, or nearly full health.

> I thought he'd get better in a day or two. I couldn't believe this was the way he was always going to be. In part I still can't believe it. But when we got home I suppose I did realise this was it. The girls were saying he might improve but that wasn't doing me any good. I must have known it wasn't to be.

Since then home life has been very difficult for her. Les can only walk a couple of steps and, at fourteen stone, he's heavy to heave around.

> Les can't listen to a television programme. He doesn't like me knitting because he doesn't like the knitting needles to click. If I'm reading he wants me to talk to him but when I talk to him he doesn't always understand.
>
> I get short-tempered with him, which isn't fair, but I feel so frustrated and stressed sometimes. I'll say to him, 'Look at that tree,' meaning outside the window, and he'll look at the other end of the room instead.

As time has passed Les has become more self-reliant. He can shave himself, wash his face, but not his body, and get on and off the toilet. He can also make a cup of tea, although he made it with cold water at first. But he's still very dependent on Pauline and this has taken its toll.

> I used to be able to sleep extremely well. Now I have nightmares about being lost, looking for something, searching for something that I can't find. I wake up

in the morning quite exhausted sometimes. I have a bad back and bad shoulders from lifting him out of the wheelchair into the car.

Pauline has tried to improve her sleep pattern.

I have a small glass of warm milk and do some reading. If things get very bad I have a relaxant tablet from my doctor and very occasionally a sleeping pill. These things help occasionally but I don't rely on them. I only take them when I feel if I don't get a good night's sleep I won't function the next day.

Pauline has refused to allow her misfortune to dominate her life completely. She could have let this happen, but instead she found a part-time job.

My work is my outside interest. It's an essential part of my life. I wasn't expected to have a career. My parents were quite Victorian in outlook and I didn't achieve much in school, but I feel I have achieved a great deal in the past few years. I've come into my own.

Through my work, I don't let Les rule my life. I have to fit in with him in lots of ways but he has to fit in with me around my work. He goes to a day-care centre two days a week and on my third working day one of our daughters looks after him. He likes it and I think it's good for him not to be stuck in the house all the time.

Once I leave him in the morning, at the day centre or at my daughter's, I don't think of him all day. I get on with work, talk to my friends. I do talk about him, of course – my life revolves around him at home. I tell them to tell me to shut up if I'm talking about him too much. But really it's a relief just to take care of myself.

This year Pauline was promoted to clerical officer in her civil service department. As well as the sense of achievement, she enjoys the company of the women she works with whom she can talk to and who encourage her to go to a keep-fit class with them. But another of her survival strategies doesn't feel so positive.

> I don't think about me. If I think about me I fall to pieces, even now. If nothing's happening with the children or the grandchildren or if Les is well and everything is ticking over nicely I can't cope. I have to think of something else other than me. I do feel very alone.
>
> Also I binge. I think a lot of carers use the comfort of having chocolates and chocolate biscuits and cakes and everything else that comes to hand. At work my eating's fine. I take in salads. But I think about my binge foods as soon as I come in through the front door. That's where the problems are.

Be Assertive

Being assertive is the key to handling stressful situations and also, in time, reducing their frequency. Assertiveness is about taking control, making decisions and advancing what you want and need while remaining aware of the wishes of others.

If our self-confidence and self-esteem are at a low level we tend to be less assertive and think what we want out of a situation isn't important. We then become more and more stressed and lose the confidence we had in situations that before hadn't been stressful or threatening.

If all around you are backlogs and your mind isn't focused on the issue in hand, it's easy to find that important decisions aren't being made. Taking control of the situation would mean dealing with one problem at a time. After all, the best way to cope with future worries is to get on with what we need to do today.

When possible it's important to learn to do things at your own pace, not at the beck and call of others. Don't be rushed into answering a question but give yourself time if that's what you want or need. Take time for yourself, too – a few minutes at regular intervals to check how you're feeling and how high your stress levels are.

Another key to behaving assertively is to try not to be too critical and aggressive towards others, as this will create a stressful atmosphere. I find it helps to remember that if something goes wrong it can nearly always be put right.

Standing back from stressful situations is also useful. Some people need high levels of stress to survive and can become addicted to that adrenalin rush. But they don't have to be the ones who create the atmosphere and set the rules – your opinion and feelings count too.

Low self-esteem is very directly bound up with assertiveness. It's difficult to say what we want if we feel we're not worth it. So try to see an error or something going wrong as forgivable or understandable or beyond your control rather than a symptom of personal deficiency.

There are many excellent books on the market about becoming more assertive. These can often be found in the women's health sections of book shops which is a shame because men, too, can find it difficult to assert themselves, as the following story illustrates.

Keith

Keith changed jobs recently and was quite shocked at how much was expected of him and also at the attitudes of his managers. He works in administration and felt he was being overloaded with work from above. He'd find one of his superiors would give him a huge chunk of business to deal with, and then before he'd had time to glance at the top sheet another of the company managers would hand him a second pile.

Keith tried to get through the work as best he could. He was new to the company and didn't like to complain or object. So he spent longer and longer sitting at his desk working too quickly and not carefully enough and feeling more and more angry and resentful.

> Looking back on it now I can't believe how much I put up with. My health started to suffer. I'd find I'd wake up with a headache in the morning and it would still be there by the time I left work, which would sometimes be eight or nine at night. For the first time in my life I'd get colds which wouldn't go away – they'd drag on for a fortnight or more.
>
> My girlfriend and I decided to go our separate ways which made me feel even more resentful towards the company. It was clear from everything she said that she wouldn't put up with me cancelling our dates any more. Work came to dominate my life completely.

Despite all the hours he was putting in, the quality of Keith's work dropped.

> Sometimes I'd complete a difficult project which they would be very pleased with but occasionally there was so much to do I'd slip up in my haste and make a mistake. Then one or other of the bosses would shout at me as if I was a child – although I would never treat a child that badly. I'm ashamed to say that the way I reacted to this was to snap at people who came to me for help. I suppose I felt I was being bullied and so I'd bully them too.

Breaking point came when one of Keith's managers, as well as criticising his work, complained about his personality and relationship with the other office staff after hearing him snap at a secretary.

> For the first time in six months I stood up for myself. I told them exactly how I was feeling, how overwhelmed I was with work from so many

different quarters, how my health and personal life had suffered.

It wasn't an easy conversation but it became clear that my managers had been unaware that I was being given work by all of them at the same time and in such great quantities. After all, I had never told them what was going on and how I felt about it. I had just presumed they knew and this was some kind of conspiracy aimed at putting me down. I know they valued the work I was doing and I think they felt quite guilty for their lack of coordination and the degree of disorganisation my story had revealed to them.

Keith met with his managers to discuss what had happened and to work out a way of easing the situation. Two months after the crisis meeting they agreed to appoint him an assistant and also paid for him to attend a time-management course to learn how to organise his day. On his own instigation, Keith also attended some assertiveness training classes run by his local authority.

It had astonished me how difficult I found it to say No when I was asked to do unreasonable amounts of work. I've learnt now that it's possible to say no without being aggressive. I've also learnt through the time-management course how to set my priorities for the day and stick to them. So if someone rings me to ask for help with the computer system – one of my responsibilities – I know now it's all right to say, 'I'm a bit tied up now. Can I call you back at three-thirty?' I can set my own agenda while listening to other people's needs at the same time and taking them into consideration.

My working day has shrunk to around eight and a half hours which is still quite long but I'm much happier, less tired and more healthy than I've been

at any time since I started in this job. I've even begun
to enjoy my work.

Let's Talk

Another excellent – and free – way of relieving stress can be
talking about what's worrying you with a member of your
family or with a friend. Talking through our emotional
difficulties can be the first step in overcoming them and it
may be that someone you know can offer you sympathy and
understanding. Of course therapists or counsellors are
available if you need a more experienced ear or want to go
into your problems in more depth, but sometimes just a talk
with someone close can help put a stressful situation into
perspective.

Often it's not the events themselves which are stressful
but how we perceive them. If our emotions have been
suppressed for a long time it can be hard to sort them
through. Talking can be the first step to releasing those
feelings. If we can't pin-point what's stressing us it can be
very difficult to deal with the stress itself. We might face the
dreaded instruction to 'Pull yourself together' from those
who also can't understand our problem and are frustrated
by that. But once we know the cause of our discontent we
can begin to deal with it.

I remember receiving a letter from a woman who'd lost
her husband a year earlier. She was feeling lonely without
him but angry at him for leaving. She felt she should be over
him and kept trying to cope with situations she believed she
ought to be able to cope with, such as going to dinner dances
on her own. The stress she was feeling at these events was
enormous. I replied to her that I could understand that she
was still grieving for her husband and it seemed to me that
she still had grieving left to do. It wasn't necessary for her to
push herself into social situations she didn't yet feel able to
cope with. She then replied to me, saying that after
receiving my letter she'd talked to her closest friends about
how she was feeling and they had said the same as I had.

They've since built up a much less pressurised social life with just a few women going out together, which my correspondent finds much easier to handle.

Talking is so straightforward and yet sometimes it can be so difficult if we dread what others will think of what we have to say. My advice would always be: if you value the person you're with and are confident of them, it's worth the risk. A problem shared is so often a problem halved, as the old saying goes.

You don't have to cope on your own and if you keep whatever's stressing you to yourself, the shame and guilt involved in keeping it hidden reinforce the problem. By talking it through you're not asking for advice or for someone else to solve all your problems, just for someone to listen to you. And if it turns out they're not sympathetic, this doesn't mean your problems aren't valid or you're not worth listening to. It might mean they can't cope with all you're telling them or that they're too wrapped up in their own problems. You will have learnt to talk to someone else next time.

If you feel you have a lot of anger inside you that's something that's good to express – not necessarily with another person but you could have a good scream and shout at home while no one else is about or bash some cushions with a tennis racket. The British aren't always very good at expressing emotions in this way but in other countries the idea is catching on. Apparently in Tokyo you can hire someone to be shouted at, from a firm which specialises in providing victims!

RELAXATION AND FUN

Talking isn't the only means of helping yourself at home. Relaxation techniques can be very useful indeed.

I learnt the ones I use on a four-and-a-half-day 'de-stressing' course many years ago. The relaxation exercises involve sitting or lying down where it's comfortable and warm, in bed maybe, and letting your body sink right down into what's supporting it, really feeling that support. Then tense and relax each part of the body in turn – ankles, thighs, trunk, arms, head and shoulders, paying special attention to the muscles likely to be tense. I tend to have tension in my shoulders and jaw, so I let my mouth fall wide open and then close it slightly, hunch my shoulders in an exaggerated fashion then let them relax. I stretch my hands and fingers like a fan and then relax them. The muscles of my forehead, too, are prone to be bunched and the skin crinkled into care lines, so I open my eyes wide, lift my brow then let the forehead relax halfway back to where it was.

By the time I have relaxed all my muscles I feel as if I'm a rag doll with no bones or muscles at all. I then think about each of my relaxed muscles individually to reinforce in my mind what they feel like when they are relaxed. This helps you to recognise and correct tiring muscular tension that develops during a stressful day.

While I'm doing this, if my mind is spinning with endless thoughts, I concentrate on one meaningless word and exclude all other thoughts from my mind which helps keep my attention focused on what's happening to my body.

Deep breathing exercises are also valuable, especially for very anxious people who breathe quickly and shallowly and so expel too much carbon dioxide gas. This can make them feel lightheaded and numb. Their muscles can go into spasm, especially their hand muscles (so much so that they find it difficult to move them). The only way the sufferer can counter this is to make a conscious effort to breathe slowly and deeply. Try sitting or lying and breathing in deeply through your nose, counting slowly to ten, holding your breath and breathing out through your mouth. Breathe normally for a few moments and then repeat this several times.

Carrying out a quick facial relaxation is also beneficial. Muscles in the face and neck are often responsible for headaches, neck and back pain. Try clenching the teeth and frowning heavily and feeling the whole of the face and neck tense up. Then let your jaw relax and your frown disappear and note how different this feels.

Learning to control the tension in muscles cuts our stress reaction right down, especially if we do this in the presence of what triggers us to be stressed – a fearsome boss at work, perhaps, or a huge spider.

Another great way to relax is to have fun – at home and at work. Laughter is an excellent treatment for stress. It reduces muscular tension, improves breathing, regulates the heart beat and pumps adrenalin and endorphins – the body's natural painkillers – into the blood stream. Group therapy in a laughter clinic opened by a psychotherapist in Birmingham is even available on the National Health Service. He had the idea after noticing that clients trying to cope with a bereavement or divorce or a similar trauma began to change the way they were looking at the problem and began to turn the corner in dealing with it when they could laugh about it.

Enjoying yourself is a great stress reliever. Playing with children, watching a favourite old comedy film, taking part in games for enjoyment and not to compete, going to one of those places you used to go years ago, such as a fair or the seaside, are all good ways of getting in touch with the fun side of life, which is easy to leave behind if we let adult responsibilities and concerns take over.

Holidays

According to *Doctor* magazine, 95 per cent of GPs have suggested at some time to patients that a holiday might do them more good than a prescription. In fact the impact of leisure on good health and in beating stress is very much at the forefront of doctors' minds.

Holidays aren't necessarily the unstressful panaceas they're made out to be however. I remember once reading a letter in the correspondence page of a newspaper which suggested that if getting into financial difficulties, meeting new people and changes are all stressful, surely holidays *add* to our problems rather than taking them away. Of course there are ways of making our holidays work with us rather than against us. If you're very stressed, a holiday that helps you to relax and rest the mind can only be of benefit. Work out what you really like to do and do it. It might be something as simple as walking or fishing or having time to write letters or a diary or listen to music. A holiday can be anything you want it to be – it doesn't have to be a trip abroad, even if that's what it's always traditionally meant for you and yours.

A recent survey showed that fewer than 25 per cent of British managerial staff routinely take their full holiday entitlement. This is despite the fact that many industrialists are aware that holidays help reduce stress-related absentee-ism – so in the long term you'll be spending less not more time at work by not taking breaks. I don't see why taking your holiday entitlement shouldn't be compulsory and I'm certain that if you didn't take your full amount your working life could become disorganised. It will almost certainly mean you're under strain. I think it's important not to wait until you're absolutely exhausted before you take a break. It's useful to have some energy to see new things and do what you enjoy rather than not being able to rise from your bed for a week. It's also important to see holidays as fun and as relaxation, not as yet another list of responsibil-ities to be worked at.

There are different theories as to how a workaholic can benefit most from a holiday. Some experts advise them to cut off completely while they're away. Others believe they need to take the shock to the system more gradually, starting off with a short break first to get used to the novelty of not working. Without this, they claim, re-entry into the real working world can be a problem. One expert was quoted as saying that going back to work after a holiday is like trying to jump on a moving train, so it's better not to slow down to walking pace but remain at a jog before you try this. For a real workaholic, a holiday can be more stressful than ordinary working life as you're not in touch with what's going on back home. On the other hand, if you're aware that you may be contacted if you stay at home – and that's the last thing you want on your week or fortnight off – then it's much more sensible to go away or at least to have a machine to answer your calls.

Holidays can also be stressful if you have over-high expectations of them – for example, if you're hoping a holiday will be an answer to all your relationship and health problems. No small break can achieve that for you. On the other hand, a holiday may be just what you need to be able to see a stressful situation from a new, refreshing perspective, as Erica found out.

Erica

Erica came home from work one day to find a surprise from her husband waiting for her. He told her their relationship was over and that he'd met someone else. She was expecting that they'd spend the evening together doing a few things in the house, having a meal, watching a video. What actually happened was that he picked up the bags he'd already packed and walked out of the door.

> The door slammed shut and I burst into tears. I was in shock, I know, but I still knew I felt devastated. I stood by the door crying and crying, my whole body was juddering. I didn't know what else to do but cry.
>
> But I also remember thinking as I sat up that whole night that I'd have to start to look after myself by myself and through my grief and my loneliness that's exactly what I did. Even at that early stage I was surprised at my inner strength. I was looking at the situation objectively and seeing that I'd played my part in the relationship breaking down. That Sam and I hadn't been getting on well for months, years even, and I'd done nothing to help move us closer together again. I just hoped our problems would magically disappear. What was good was that I could see that this disaster in my life

wasn't something that had just happened to me. I'd played my part. Thinking like that felt better than filling my head with bitterness and cynicism.

Erica found a great deal of support from those around her.

Lots of people were great, including my grandmother and a particular male friend who had just split up from his partner. I was also very surprised at the support I received from work. I'd presumed they wouldn't be interested in my personal problems but they were very concerned and asked if I was seeing a counsellor, if I had a good lawyer and if I was OK for money.

In the first couple of days of the split I was supposed to see a friend. She heard the news on the grapevine and rang me and said, 'I guess you are going to be preoccupied and you won't want to see me now so I won't call you for a couple of weeks.' But I said, 'I would really like it if you did call me,' and she did and it was really good to talk to her. Although we hadn't been that close beforehand she turned out to be a really strong support.

I didn't realise it at the time but now I see that was one of the ways I dealt with the stress of the situation – which would have been unbearable if I hadn't shared it – by talking to other people about it.

Talking was one of Erica's coping mechanisms. Her other was, maybe more surprisingly, to go on holiday.

I decided to go alone. I thought, 'I've got to learn to be on my own.' I was meant to be going with Sam but obviously that had all been cancelled so then I started looking around for someone else to go with. Then suddenly I started getting excited and interested in the idea of being by myself and not having to organise myself around anyone else. I thought, 'I want to be on my own.' I didn't see it as second best but as something I'd chosen to do.

Before I went away I was very jumpy. I didn' settle at all. Sometimes I wasn't eating and I was smoking like a trooper. I lived on cigarettes and alcohol – not half a bottle of whisky a night or anything, but for me I was drinking a lot. I always smoke in times of stress but because Sam had never liked me smoking being able to do this was a sign of freedom. Now there was nobody to criticise me – and nobody for me to imagine being critical. At other times I was over-eating, binging a lot. I'd wake in the middle of the night, turning things over in my head, terrible, tortured conversations I'd been having with Sam over the phone, or fears about my future on my own.

This was Erica's state of mind before her holiday. No wonder she was looking forward to it.

On the holiday itself I did very, very little. I just sat quietly and watched the world go by. Sometimes I didn't go to bed till three in the morning. Sometimes I'd go to sleep in the evening, wake up in the middle of the night and read until I was tired again. That was OK too – anything I wanted to do was OK. I remember that I didn't cry that much on holiday – it felt as if somehow I was giving my emotions a rest.

I had a wonderful time. It wasn't fun in the sense of telling jokes and dancing till dawn but it was very enjoyable. I can't remember this very clearly but I don't even think I missed Sam very much. The only time I thought of him a lot was at meal times. Then I'd remember that when I'd been away with him food was a big deal for us. We'd spend ages deciding when and where to eat. It was quite a focus of the day. Then we'd see what each other was choosing and eating. When I was on my own meals became perfunctory, just food.

Erica's holiday helped her to rediscover what she liked to do and what she wanted to do.

When I got back I saw Sam and said I was prepared to have a go at working out our relationship. He said he wasn't. I realised straight away that the best thing for me was not to have any more contact with him and that's what I told him. I had to learn to live life by myself. I knew I could. The holiday had shown me that. I realised it would have been more and more painful seeing him. My wounds couldn't have healed. As long as I wanted our relationship to start again and he didn't we could never be equal. We had been having good conversations, getting on better than ever in fact, and yet he didn't want to have a relationship with me again. He still had another girlfriend. We had been meeting up, talking, and he was going back to someone else. Our meetings would always start with a fight, then we'd become friends, then he'd go home to a different place with a different woman waiting for him there.

I realised I was going to have to tell him our meetings would have to end. The night before I did this I cried and cried. I knew the sense of loss would be so great. The next morning I called him, told him, hung up the phone, ran to the loo and cried. I thought to myself, 'What would my fairy godmother say to me now?' She would say, 'You've made a very difficult and painful decision and this is releasing you from a very difficult and painful situation. He can't hurt you any more.'

On the holiday, with my routine taken away and all other people I knew taken away, I'd recovered a sense of myself and who I was, what I needed and what I didn't need. It was a difficult decision not to

> see Sam because I really wanted him. I wanted to
> have things as they had been.

This was another turning point for Erica. She started to recognise the good things in her life. She had a new flat to herself which she enjoyed and she started to realise how stressful it had been living in a relationship that was breaking down.

> I'd coped with that by denying it. I knew Sam was
> unhappy. He'd told me he was re-evaluating his life
> and I didn't ask him if this re-evaluation involved
> me. Instead we just went to a party and blanked it
> out. I didn't want to know.
>
> Now I was feeling the positive stress that comes
> with change. Exciting things were happening in my
> life. I joined a gym, I was looking really good, my
> skin had an amazing glow to it. Someone said to me,
> 'You should get divorced more often!'

Erica and Sam didn't talk for a week until one evening he called her saying he'd been thinking about them getting back together again.

> I didn't leap up and down and say, 'Yes, please.' I just
> asked him some questions and then on my sugges-
> tion we went to see a counsellor together.
>
> When we got back together I sobbed hysterically
> and told him it was awful. I must have been denying
> to myself quite how awful I felt when we were apart
> and how angry and sad I felt about him finding
> another woman. But altogether I'm proud of the
> way I handled it. I never once said to myself, 'You
> should be over this by now.' I imagine if I had things
> would have become much more stressful again
> because I'd have been trying to avoid what I was
> feeling.

Keep Fit

Keeping fit can mean having fun, relaxing and pushing yourself to your healthy limits all at the same time. As well as giving you a general sense of well-being, exercise uses up stress hormones which otherwise stay in the blood keeping us tense. Swimming is a natural massage and problems can float away in a pool. Added to this, healthy tired muscles have a calming effect and can help raise self-esteem. Thirty minutes of exercise three times a week is a good target to reach to keep your body and mind in condition.

Teresa

One young woman I've heard from had to find a way of coping with the very stressful situation in which she found herself when she and her husband and their two boys had moved to a new town. She realised that she needed some time to herself and found that an aerobics class was the way she could have those couple of hours a week away from her family and all the changes she was having to face in her life.

> For me aerobics is a great way of being on my own which sometimes I feel I desperately need. It also helps me let off steam and get rid of any angry feelings I have. I just get in that hall and work away like mad to the music and come out feeling that I have so much more energy than I could have ever imagined at the time I dragged myself into my leotard!

Teresa has many stressful situations to cope with all at the same time. The move was the result of a promotion for her husband Danny, which meant more responsibility and longer working hours for him. She too moved to a new job in a field she'd never worked in before. Matthew, who's eight, had to get used to a new school and three-year-old Gavin started going to a new nursery. Everything was new.

The move has unsettled us more than I ever imagined. It's worst first thing in the morning. Matthew won't get out of bed, Gavin won't get dressed, Matthew won't eat his breakfast. Then I find out Matthew hasn't told me about things he needs for school – his PE clothes which are still dirty and in his bag from last time is a great example – or he tells me he hasn't done his homework. All this time I'm trying to get ready for work and I'm thinking, 'I can only give them so much. At some point I have to tell them, No, no no.' Then there's a temper tantrum and they start shouting or I end up shouting at them which leaves me feeling horrible.

If this all happens when we're out of the house I'm aware of people thinking, 'Oh God, what a terrible mother. Why can't she control her children?' and I'm thinking, 'Oh, no.'

So compared with all of this an exercise class feels like heaven. It's my way of relaxing. Surprisingly it can feel more relaxing and be better at removing stress than slumping in an armchair at home. Afterwards I might have a sauna and then I just lie there and forget about everything. I've worked through my pent-up frustration and then I just float away for another twenty minutes. Fabulous!

Teresa knows she has a long way to go before her life feels more in control. The family's still coming to terms with its new location. What she and her husband aren't doing is going out as a couple without the children, which she feels would be beneficial for both of them.

Aerobics is my way of remembering that I'm me as well as a mother and wife. I think me and Danny need to remember we're real people as well as parents. We never seem to have time for ourselves as a couple. I'd love to get away without the kids but I couldn't do it. I'd feel guilty because my mum left

me when I was very little for a few years and I
remember how terrible I felt. I was with my
grandmother who loved me but I wanted to be with
my mother and I swore I'd never leave my children,
even for a couple of days. Now I think it might do
me and Danny some good to get away and have
time to ourselves, and so I'm trying to talk myself
into it. That would really help us put our pressures
and problems right behind us and give us a bit of an
energy booster.

FOOD

For anyone trying to lead a less stressed life, healthy eating
is essential. A poor diet and insufficient vitamins can be a
factor in increasing stress levels and can lead to the body
coping much less efficiently with stress.

Eating regular meals is one important rule, as is cutting
down on refined convenience foods. Wholefoods and fresh
fruit and vegetables in their place are ideal, along with small
quantities of animal products including eggs and dairy
produce and fish high in calcium. Aim for foods rich in
vitamins, minerals and fibre and low in added chemicals, fats
and too much sugar. Don't drink too much tea or coffee
apart from herbal teas.

Foods rich in magnesium and zinc, including nuts, soya
beans, beetroot and peaches, are recommended to help build
up against the ill-effects of stress, as are sunflower and
sesame seeds, brown rice, bran, wheat germ, brewers' yeast,
onions and oysters. I'm a firm believer that a relaxed
breakfast is a calm and nourishing way to start the day and
will help keep stress at bay. It's also an idea to spend ten
minutes or so before a main meal sitting quietly, possibly
with a pre-dinner drink, to allow the muscles to relax and set
the stomach up to function well during the meal. Herbal
camomile tea is another good way to stave off the gastric
disorders brought on by tension which can be so painful and

unpleasant. Others include eating your meal at a table, certainly away from your desk while you're at work, and always eating slowly, chewing well.

My postbag tells me many people find supplements a useful addition to a diet and these can be found in any chemist or health shop. B vitamins play an important role in the production of anti-stress hormones, with B6 particularly useful. Vitamins C and E are also useful and Ginseng may be a bonus too.

Health shops sell many different natural tranquillisers – you may find a special section of various brands in your local store. As with conventional tranquillisers, these won't remove underlying causes of stress but you may find they help you to relax, sleep and feel better equipped to face some of the issues that are troubling you. Homoeopathic and herbal remedies which can help too are covered in the next chapter (see page 101).

SELF-HELP WHILE DRIVING

I've decided to include a special section in this chapter on driving as this can be a very stressful activity. I've heard one expert say that driving in a busy city leads to as much stress as motor racing or parachuting, with increases to the heart rate of 120 to 180 beats per minute. Motoring organisations have many suggestions on how to cut down on stress behind the wheel, which almost inevitably means cutting down on accidents at the same time and that has to be a good thing.

Surveys show that it's more stressful driving after work, when the day has got to you, than it is earlier in the day. Other drivers' behaviour is said to be the biggest source of stress, ahead of road conditions and attempts to keep appointments. Domestic rows before driving, illness, drinking alcohol, lethargy, aggression, loss of sleep and night driving all add to stress according to the Institute of Advanced Motorists.

Blood pressure and adrenalin levels can rise just by being exposed to the noise of traffic so think what sitting in a jam can do. Breaking down on motorways is very anxiety provoking, especially for women.

So for less stressful, and so less accident-prone, motoring, driving organisations suggest:

- Making sure you and your passengers are comfortable before you set off.
- Planning your journey in advance, knowing where you're going, knowing distances, routes and landmarks. Leaving plenty of time for hold-ups. Try to avoid rush hours.
- Never driving for more than eight hours a day, with a break after three at the wheel. It's best to have a passenger who can take over the driving from time to time.
- Trying some breathing exercises, and exercises for your head and shoulders while at the wheel when safely stopped.
- Not taking any drugs which impair driving, nor having heavy meals or alcohol before or during your trip.
- Driving in daylight when possible and sleeping well beforehand.
- Making sure the car is well ventilated. Remember to do this if you're using your heater in cold weather as this can make you drowsy.
- Listening to the car radio or music which can reduce stress and anxiety.
- Carrying spare petrol and being confident about the mechanical condition of the car, the pressure in the tyres and the oil and water levels. Don't forget to check the spare tyre. Keep a note of emergency numbers for the breakdown services. If you're a woman driving on your own, make sure you tell the breakdown services this on the phone and stay in your car while you wait for them to arrive.
- Checking in the driving mirror when you're stuck in a traffic jam to see if your jaw's set tight, your eyes are

screwed up or your knuckles are white. If this is a description of you, you're experiencing useless and unnecessary stress at the wheel. Try those breathing and relaxation exercises.

• Driving calmly and non-competitively.

STRESS – WHAT NOT TO DO

When stressed lots of people turn to alcohol to help them through. Millions of others light up a cigarette. Some take illegal drugs. Many women, especially, binge on comfort foods. But none of these are healthy, and nor are they successful ways of relieving stress.

The initial numbing effect of alcohol, for example, is very pleasing but after this has worn off too much alcohol increases symptoms of depression and anxiety. Drinking, like taking tranquillisers, can help to hide the stress symptoms but does not get rid of the stress. Of course, drinking in moderation is fine and can even be beneficial, but drinking to escape from problems just brings on more of them.

Alcohol isn't the only culprit. Too much caffeine, too much nicotine and the long-term use of tranquillisers or sleeping pills may at first seem to help but in the end they interfere with the body's natural ability to control stress.

Tobacco and alcohol also prevent Vitamins B1, B2 and B6 and Vitamin C being absorbed by the body. One figure I've read is that for every cigarette you smoke, 25mg of Vitamin C is used up – the quantity of this vital vitamin found in a small orange.

I've also never heard anyone who gorges themselves on more food than they can comfortably eat feel good about themselves, their body or their dietary habits. And that's a very stressful way to live.

Molly

Molly's problem, since she was a teenager, was drinking. It had always been her answer to stress of any form. Then five months ago she made the decision to join Alcoholics Anonymous.

> At the time I made the decision to stop drinking life had become almost unmanageable. My relationships were in a bad way. I'd continually get into situations with people I regretted – especially with men – but everything seemed to be out of my control. When I decided to quit I thought, 'This will be really good. Now I'll be able to tackle my problems in my relationships and my behaviour.' But after a week, to my astonishment, the problems ceased to exist. My drinking had been the cause.

Molly found that situations she had been drinking to escape from, such as people looking down on her, didn't exist in her sober world. She had been trying to escape from a mirage.

She told me how she came from a family of heavy drinkers.

> I was drinking really heavily by the time I was fifteen. That's how I had a good time. My social life revolved around the pub. Everyone would get drunk and so would I.
>
> My self-esteem was low and I was pathologically shy. If I opened my mouth in public I thought everyone would think I was stupid, but once I had a drink I'd think I was the bee's knees and really witty. I lost my inhibitions. Drinking helped me not to care about other people. It dulled my senses. It made me think I was right and everyone else was wrong. And it enabled me to deceive myself to the point where I could no longer make any claim to having much of a grip on reality. If a man looked at me I would get

so paranoid and stressed out. I'd think about how I was going to cope with rejection – when nothing had even happened.

I'd drink anything and everything. If I was having a quiet evening at home with a friend, we'd get through two or three bottles of wine between us. And if we'd come across any drugs we'd take them too for the novelty and the different kick. Sometimes when I took drugs it was a complete lucky dip. I'd think, 'I don't know how this drug will make me feel, up or down, but it will make me feel different from how I'm feeling now and that's the main thing.' I was playing Russian Roulette with my emotions.

Molly knew her dependence on alcohol was extremely stressful but she liked that as part of her image. 'I thought stress was glamorous, "See me, I'm really stressed because my life's so full." I'd look at the next week in my diary and it would be all full up.' But her health was suffering.

I'd ricochet between insomnia and lethargy. It was very difficult to know if it was the stress or the alcohol. I had upset stomachs – that could have been either the stress or the alcohol, as well. I suppose the whole thing is cumulative.

First the drink would be numbing then I'd be completely anaesthetised. After that I'd be either going up or coming down. In that state I'd sit and drink strong black coffee with two sugars, one cup after another which would give me the shakes.

I'd take pride in the fact that I could drink lots of people under the table, then could go into work after two hours' sleep. I took that as a symbol of being able to stay in control but what I was actually doing was stressing my body and my mind with drugs and alcohol, cigarettes and caffeine. It does you in physically, mentally, emotionally, spiritually.

Your body suffers, your relationships suffer, you forget who you are. I call it holistic self-destruction.

I'd start drinking earlier and earlier and earlier. I'd wait for the shop to be open so I could buy a bottle of red wine and have my first taste of the day. I'd expect it to calm me down but instead it would wind me up even more. I realised I was destroying myself but I just kept going. It was all I knew to do.

Molly changed course after a very frightening incident happened to her. There was a break-in at her home while she was in bed one night, and for half an hour she seriously believed she was going to die.

That incident with the burglar made me realise that life is very sweet. No matter how bad it is, when there's a moment when you think it's going to be taken away from you it suddenly becomes pretty good. I realised then that I was killing myself, deadening myself. I looked at the mess my life was in – everything from my bank account to my wardrobe to my relationships. When I looked round for the culprit it wasn't hard to find her.

She joined Alcoholics Anonymous and they proved to be a huge support.

I can't begin to describe the support I found there. I never had anywhere I could just go and be before. I finally found somewhere I belonged. I'd sit and listen to other people relating their stories and I often thought how closely they related to mine.

CONVENTIONAL AND ALTERNATIVE TREATMENT

However clearly we recognise that stress is causing us problems, and may be damaging our health, and however hard we try to alter our lifestyles to bring less tension and more calmness into our lives, sometimes it simply isn't possible to deal with all the causes and symptoms by ourselves. Indeed, the very symptoms that stress can bring, including listlessness and a lack of energy, may be some of the reasons why alone we don't feel strong and purposeful enough to make the changes we need.

Often I've found people not wanting to face up to the stress they're under and the effect it's having on their personalities, their health, their relationships, their work and their play. They may feel it's a sign of weakness to want to seek help, that they should be able to manage by themselves. 'Macho' messages about not showing weaknesses and needs still seem to persist.

For me, the opposite is true. I believe it's a sign of strength to overcome those messages and allow yourself to look for and accept care and advice from others.

There has been a phenomenal increase in the popularity of various alternative therapies and medicines in recent years and many of them can be excellent when it comes to stress relief and treatment. More conventionally, a common first stop for those seeking help is the family doctor and this is where I'll begin.

YOUR DOCTOR

I remember clearly from my days as a GP how often and how quickly the word 'stress' leapt to mind as soon as some of my patients began to describe their symptoms or their state of mind.

If you do want to see your doctor, and if there is an appointment system, try to make an appointment at a less busy time for the GP. It might be useful to take in some notes of what you want to tell him or her in case you feel nervous or rushed once you're inside the surgery and in case you're worried you'll forget to mention one of your symptoms and fears. However, try to keep concise and to the point – no doctor has limitless time. It might also be an idea to jot down some of the things the doctor says to you to be sure you'll remember any reassurance and practical suggestions you're given. Some doctors will welcome a tape recorder so that you can remind yourself of what was said as many times as you like.

Many patients who suffer from stress expect to be prescribed tranquillisers to help them cope – the National Health Service often seems to be based on feeling bad and being given a cure. Yet a doctor can and should do much more than just write out a prescription. Over the years GPs have found themselves labelled with a reputation for doling out tranquillisers without a second thought to anyone suffering from stress who walks through the surgery door. Personally I think this reputation is far from universally deserved, and one particular case which came from my postbag seems a good way to illustrate both this and the help and support a doctor can give without medication being involved.

Linda
Linda is thirty and has a highly pressured job, working in administration for a clothing factory. Her stress levels only presented her with problems which seemed insurmountable when her mother, depressed after a car accident which left her confined to a wheelchair, ended her own life.

'I went back to work immediately after the funeral,' she remembers.

There was a huge pile of papers in my in-tray which would normally have given me a fair amount of anxiety but they didn't even bother me. I couldn't do anything with them. I just sat there. I did nothing except every couple of hours I'd go outside and walk up and down the road, then go into a café and have a cup of tea. Then I'd go into work again and look at the papers again and decide there was nothing I could do with them.

Linda is describing a fairly typical shock reaction to a highly traumatic life event.

I felt like my brain was full of cotton wool and I told my boss I couldn't do anything. Luckily he was sympathetic and said he'd be worried about me if I *could* do anything. The weekend came and I wandered around going from café to café, reading, drinking tea and smoking. I wanted people around me but I didn't want to talk to any of them. It felt as if I was living in a different world from everybody else.

I struggled through the next few weeks but by then work had become very heavy and very stressful. I had to try to concentrate on getting the job done and this left me no time at all to think about my mum. But the feelings would come anyway. I'd think about her on the bus to work and in between meetings, but I wouldn't let myself cry. I didn't think it would be right to come to work blubbing.

Linda couldn't keep the tears away for ever. They broke through when she wasn't expecting an outburst – on the way back from the supermarket on Saturday.

I started crying and crying. I had to stop the car and just sit by the side of the road and cry. It was a bit of a relief, but generally I didn't talk about my grief and looking back that must have left me very stressed. I certainly remember not sleeping well and waking up with really bad aches and pains in my joints at four in the morning.

Realising that this was all connected with her mother's sudden suicide, Linda knew she needed some help to come to terms with what had happened and also to help her work out how to cope with a stressful job and a torrent of emotions she didn't want to release. She made an appointment with her GP.

My doctor is very good and has often been supportive in the past, giving me time even when there's been a bit of a queue in the waiting room. She talked with me about everything that had happened. She said, 'You're not grieving, you haven't given yourself a chance to grieve.' It sounds obvious now, but I really hadn't thought of it in such simple terms. By the end of my appointment I was in tears and she told me I had to have some time off work and gave me a sick note.

Part of me heard her say I had to have the time off, the other part thought I was indispensable and couldn't possibly not go in to that ever growing pile of papers. So I left the surgery to drive to a meeting that I'd rescheduled so I could fit in my doctor's appointment. But no sooner had I started to drive when I had to stop the car. I just couldn't stop crying. I turned round, came home and cried for two days, staring into space and crying. I didn't answer the phone. I can't remember if I ate anything or not, I only remember crying.

At the weekend I went round to some friends for a meal. It was a struggle to be with people and make conversation with them. After the lunch I felt sick and ill. I fell asleep on their sofa but when I woke I felt much worse and was very sick. They brought

> me home and called the doctor. I've never felt so ill.
> I was so ill I couldn't open my mouth to speak.
>   I actually felt I was dying. I felt so weak I was sure
> I was going to slip away. I did feel it was a shame
> because I'm only thirty but I accepted I wasn't going
> to survive. The doctor came out to me and said it
> was a culmination of all the stress I'd been under
> and that I had to stay in bed for a few days. I
> continued to be sick the whole of that night and the
> next day. Then I stayed in bed for two days, worked
> at home for two and then went back in.

Linda had taken some time off, although her need to
work had stopped her from staying away from the office for
too long.

> Now I think back to it and wonder how I coped with
> only one week off sick in total for all that time. It
> seems incredible. I'm very relieved that my doctor
> gave me that advice and my respect for her views
> allowed me to take in what she was saying although
> part of me felt work couldn't cope without me.
>   Still now I have huge bursts of grief. I cry and cry
> and I'm amazed there's so much of it still there.
> Afterwards I feel full of energy. Now I try to face
> any painful feelings as they come up – I think if I can
> face them now they're not going to come back later.
> At the time I put all my energy into being able to
> cope and there was no energy left for letting all
> those feelings out.

So, rather than prescribing tranquillisers which would
have merely postponed the emotional stress in Linda's case,
her doctor persuaded her to make time to process her
feelings and relieve the stress they were causing. The doctor
was also able to suggest further help because Linda confided
in her that she still felt she was going to die.

I'd go to work on the bus thinking about my own funeral, about the people who'd come and how sad they'd be. It was just like watching an event unfolding. I had no control over it – I wasn't even that bothered. I had a recurring dream that I died in a car crash. For a month I even stopped driving apart from when it was absolutely necessary. In the dream I'd be driving on my own, it was winter with no leaves on the trees and the car went into a spin at sixty miles per hour. My doctor said she didn't know what the dream meant but she was sure it didn't mean I was about to die. She suggested a psychotherapist who might be able to help and I started seeing her. The therapist confirmed the dream wasn't about my death. She told me she felt the car represented my mother and the car crash was a representation of the way that so dramatically and finally our relationship had terminated. She also helped me work through my bereavement in other ways.

I still feel alone – totally alone in a way I've never felt before. But without the support I've had directly and indirectly from my doctor I know I wouldn't have coped as well as I have.

I feel Linda's doctor was absolutely right to act as counsellor and advisor and not to prescribe tranquillising drugs. She saw that Linda's need was to talk, to let go of her feelings and release some of the pain and grief which was building up inside her. Like many doctors she could recommend a professional counsellor who could give Linda more time and more expert care. My feeling, in any case, is that tranquillisers don't help at a time of bereavement. However many pills are taken, the individual is still left with the bereavement and months of pretty severe distress. It's unavoidable.

A good doctor – and Linda's sounds just that – should allow you time to talk, or at least check that you have someone you can confide in. It's very important that when you're leaving the surgery you feel you have been listened to and taken seriously. If you have physical symptoms that you're worried about – and which are adding to your stress – ask about them. If your heart seems to be beating rapidly does that mean you might have palpitations? Might you be in danger of a heart attack? Your doctor should be able to put your mind at rest on both counts. Try not to see your fears and worries as too trivial to bring to the doctor's attention. This will just mean they stay to plague you after your trip to the surgery is over.

You may be prescribed tranquillisers or anti-depressants – after all, anti-anxiety drugs are the most frequently prescribed drugs in the Western world. I think it's important that the decision about whether you take medication for stress is reached by both you and your doctor. If you're the one who's very keen for tablets ask yourself if there are problems in your life you don't want to face – you'd rather block them off in some way in the hope that they'll vanish of their own accord, which they won't. If your doctor is suggesting them, check that you feel you've been given enough time to explore alternatives with him or her and that you don't feel you're being fobbed off with a piece of paper. Every doctor has a different view about how best to treat stress and it's important that you feel your doctor's view is the same as your own. If you feel you need to talk, it's important to say so. This also gives the doctor a chance to consider whether a counsellor should be recommended.

Tranquillisers are far from a dream answer for the treatment of stress. They can be addictive and can also numb good feelings as well as bad. I tend to feel that tranquillisers, which block the body's anxiety receptors, can cause many more problems than they solve unless they're prescribed for very short periods of time. (There are fewer problems with taking anti-depressants, see pages 74–5.)

Having said all this, I do feel that prescribing tranquillisers on a short-term basis has its uses when treatment for stress is required. I remember one young man writing to me – his unhappy marriage had broken up and he'd just found out he was going to lose his home. Other sides of his life were going well, he had a good job and a reasonable income. He needed to tackle the problems this crisis in his life was throwing at him but he found he couldn't. He was suffering from tension headaches and recurrent insomnia, yet was not interested in any method of dealing with his stress such as meditation. Usually a confident person, he now felt as if he was falling to pieces – he couldn't even make a list of things he needed to do. In his case, a course of tranquillisers for a couple of weeks would probably help him get through the practicalities he has to deal with at this very difficult time in his life.

I'm not talking here about the major tranquillisers used for patients suffering from mental illness under the care of a psychiatrist. Benzodiazepines such as Valium or Librium can be useful for those of us who are not mentally ill but for whom life's circumstances have reached such a pitch that we seem to be turning into a wriggling mass of nerves.

The dangers with tranquillisers come from misuse and from using them for longer than a couple of weeks. Your doctor should monitor you closely if you are taking a course. Side-effects can include depression, nausea, dizziness, drowsiness and tiredness, personality changes, loss of appetite, diarrhoea and aches in the joints and muscles. There can also be occasional menstrual problems, weight gain and skin rashes. Accidents are also more likely and driving can be impaired. As with alcohol, you may feel better very quickly because of the anaesthetic effect but, also as with alcohol, in your day-to-day life you'll function much worse. It's likely that you'll be advised not to drink alcohol during a course and tranquillisers should not be taken in early or late pregnancy or when breastfeeding.

If someone is feeling so depressed as to be thinking of taking their own life, I see anti-depressants as, in the main, a much safer medicine. They won't solve the problems that led to the depression but they are non-addictive and they can help the sufferer to cope with depression.

Someone who's severely depressed will have physiological changes to his or her body, it is thought due to a depletion of neurotransmitters – the chemical messengers in the brain which carry messages from one nerve cell to another. This can bring aches and pains to the body, an inability to sleep and other very unpleasant symptoms. Anti-depressants restore the ability of neurotransmitters to work efficiently and so the depressed person should feel physically better and thus more able to cope with their mental pain.

Drugs such as beta-blockers may also be prescribed to patients under great stress. They have a lower potential for abuse and help to reduce physical symptoms such as palpitations, sweating and shaking, and produce calm by slowing the heart rate. But they do have less of a psychological effect and with these drugs too there are side-effects. For someone with a tendency to asthma, for example, beta-blockers can provoke an attack.

Maybe as many as a quarter of a million people have been dependent on tranquillisers. Some estimates have been higher. Dependence comes because the body adapts when it takes in the substance which it doesn't naturally use – just as it adapts when it takes in alcohol or nicotine or caffeine. The body's tolerance to the substance can increase and so more is needed to produce the same effect. The body relies on it to function and when the substance is withdrawn – completely or, preferably, gradually – the dependent person feels ill. Stress levels can become higher at this point in the short term, and some dependents have taken anti-depressants while withdrawing from tranquillisers.

Having said this, I feel that many who could benefit from short-term tranquilliser use now don't because when they hear the word 'tranquilliser' they also hear the word 'addiction'. There have been horror stories, and I'm sure there has been over-prescribing, especially before the addictive nature of the drugs was fully appreciated, but tranquillisers do have a role to play in calming the anxious and relieving insomnia. (Anxiety and stress are the biggest causes of insomnia as they keep the mind so preoccupied it keeps reactivating itself and the sufferer lies awake, tortured by his or her thoughts and unable to fall into a restful sleep.)

Doctors sometimes say that it's not they who are so keen on prescribing tranquillisers but the patients who feel they want to leave with a prescription in their hands. It's an unofficial tradition of the National Health Service that you go to the doctor and leave with a piece of paper.

But with stress the answer is never that simple and straightforward. What I feel is more important is that you are able to talk to your doctor about what's worrying you and that he or she can counsel you about some of your medical fears. Doctors often have to reassure their patients – after a thorough investigation – that palpitations, headaches, dizziness and indigestion need not indicate heart disorder, a brain tumour, stomach cancer or some other dreaded disease. While it seems logical to suppose that physical symptoms have a physical cause and cure, in fact they can all be brought on by stress and anxiety. Sometimes a doctor's explanation of why the body is reacting in this way and a bit of reassurance may be enough to prevent the symptoms recurring. Understanding how your nerves can cause such a range of symptoms is often enough to remove the fear of them and this can be the best cure of all.

As I've already mentioned, if the problems are more widespread or deep-rooted your doctor can point you in the direction of a counsellor, psychotherapist or psychologist who can give you more time and attention and who has the right training and skills to help you with what's stressing you. Some GPs' surgeries have counsellors who work in association with them on the NHS. Helping sufferers to identify their fears, work through them and feel more positive about themselves can in time be very successful. It's important that you feel comfortable talking to your doctor. If you feel your GP is looking awkward as you speak of your concerns or appears uncomfortable at you crying or showing other emotions, it may be that a change of doctor is what you need more than a packet of pills. Tranquillisers may remove some of the symptoms of the stress you're suffering but they can't remove the cause. Only by examining your life and your problems can you begin to do that and you'll need to feel confident that your GP has a sympathetic ear.

It may be that you prefer to see a woman doctor, or that you prefer to see a man. It may be that you wish to keep to the same doctor in a large practice rather than take pot-luck on whoever has a free appointment. Allowing yourself these choices is a significant step in taking control of your health care. And these days changing from a doctor you're not happy with to a new one – maybe one recommended by a friend or neighbour – is a very simple procedure.

If you do decide with your doctor that tranquillisers would help you cope with stress, check exactly what's being prescribed and why. If you feel at all anxious about the drugs then tell this to your doctor or you will simply leave the surgery with something else to feel stressed about. Ask any questions you may have about the effects of the drugs, about any side-effects and about how long they will take to work. But, as I've already said, tranquillisers don't solve the underlying causes of stress and anxiety, and because of this and the risk of dependence they tend to be prescribed only in the short term for cases of extreme distress. There are many other ways of getting help if stress becomes too big a problem in your life.

Counselling and Psychotherapy

This is perhaps one of the most in-depth methods of treating stress – guiding you as you look at the roots of discontent and tension. When self-esteem is low and you seem not to be in charge of your life, the help of an expert in examining the negative patterns of behaviour which we all have, and looking at the choices we can make instead, is often invaluable.

It's quite difficult in a few words to give a sense of the difference between the kinds of help available. With counselling, which for a private session will probably cost around £30–£40 an hour, you sit face to face with your counsellor and talk to him or her about what's troubling you. Counselling helps mainly with short-term problems and you should receive a genuine, empathic and non-judgemental response from your counsellor. With psycho-therapy, which will cost up to £60 a session, you can expect to deal more intensively with longer term problems, looking at some of the reasons for them in your past. With behavioural or humanistic psychotherapy you will probably sit opposite your therapist and, again, you can expect to do most of the talking. You may also play a more physical part, using Gestalt techniques such as hitting cushions with a bat to release anger. With psychoanalysis you will pay anything up to £100 per session. Analysis concentrates more on dreams and your childhood, looking at both your conscious and your unconscious life. While it is not an answer to short-term problems, it may have long-term benefits though I believe it takes much longer to achieve these.

Counselling and sometimes the other forms of help can be available through your GP, as I've mentioned above. Some doctors operate stress clinics where counsellors are available or a doctor can refer you to clinical psychology services at local hospitals (clinical psychologists are familiar with stress management techniques). Many companies offer stress counselling to employees. Counsellors can also be contacted through the British Association for Counsel-ling, whose address can be found at the back of this book and whose members include such organisations as the West-minster Pastoral Foundation and Relate (which used to be the Marriage Guidance Council) as well as private individual counsellors.

Some people who feel they are suffering from stress are reluctant to see their doctor about it because they don't want it on a medical certificate or in their medical records. Many see it as admitting to a psychological problem or a mental illness, when it's just everyday stress, which doesn't need the attentions of a psychiatrist, just a shoulder to cry on, an understanding ear and some well-chosen words of advice. 'They're not ill, they're just going through a difficult time,' says Caroline Raymond, an experienced stress consultant.

She agrees that embarrassment about admitting to a problem with stress is one reason people stay away from seeking help. 'Many feel others will think they're weak and can't cope – and they're right. There is a lot of hostility to stress. This is particularly true in the workplace where by admitting to stress an individual may run greater risks of losing his or her job. Stress must be the one thing that, although we don't want to have it, we sometimes get a sense of relief by knowing that someone also has it. The relief comes from knowing, "It's not just me!"'

Caroline says her stress counselling often comes into play when people don't recognise their own limitations – for example, perhaps they're in a situation at work which is too much for them. As a visiting stress consultant at their workplace she will help them determine where the stress is coming from and, if the problem area lies within her expertise, she may deal with it. If not, she will refer them to someone specialising in the necessary area, such as a relaxation therapist, an assertiveness trainer, a redundancy counsellor, a bereavement counsellor or a specialist in sex therapy. She believes that although for many the workplace can be a highly frustrating and accordingly stressful place, in reality stress comes from both the individual's working and domestic life.

Caroline is the founder of Stress in Perspective, an organisation offering sensible straightforward advice and guidance on the reduction of negative stress. Together with other professionals from the stress world, she offers organisations a service geared to their specific needs. This can take the form of a full-day course or a more in-depth training programme.

The areas Caroline specialises in include relationship problems and mid-life crises, but during her years as a consultant she's witnessed the stresses which have led people of all ages to her door.

'These days young people are under a high level of stress. Not only do they often have problems finding jobs but many of the shyer young people find modern sexual codes very difficult to cope with.

'Then there are those who are older and find they're not achieving what they wanted to and realise they may no longer have the time to do so. They may have married young and joined the roller coaster, doing all the things their parents wanted them to do. Then they wake up at thirty-five thinking, "I don't want to be doing this." A lot of people are reviewing how they operate and want to make changes. For example, both men and women, at this stage, may question their sexual needs thinking, "I don't really want to sleep with this person any longer." This can be very stressful for them and, of course, for their partners.

'For the elderly there's the stress of sometimes being physically very cold, of travelling being more difficult, health less good and the loneliness of old age.'

Loneliness is a major stressor for all ages, adds Caroline. 'We need to feel a sense of belonging. For example, in the past this was, in many cases, provided by the Church and close-knit family communities – both sadly becoming things of the past. Loneliness can even manifest itself within marriages where the partners though not wanting to be together cannot find the strength to overcome all the financial, emotional and social implications of parting. And although much more accepted these days for many gay people there also can be tremendous loneliness.'

Caroline believes the improvement in world communications – that we can turn the television on and witness people starving to death – stresses many of us, as does the amount of decision-making we have to do in our modern lives. Counselling, she says, can help us see things in perspective and make our choices, and help us grow and so get out of life all we can.

Eleanor

Someone who feels she's benefited greatly from counselling and psychotherapy is Eleanor, a twenty-two-year-old who's just left college with a good degree. She's bright and very contented with what she's achieved in her years of education, but she's achieved this with the help of counsellors who gave her advice and support as she coped with a crisis in the middle of her studies.

> My first year went OK. But when I went back to college after the summer holidays I started to get depressed. I began to feel very lacking in confidence and very anxious about writing essays. Making notes was fine but when it actually came to trying to put something down on paper I felt I couldn't do it. I would write and rewrite and rewrite. I'd do a paragraph and instead of moving on I'd try to perfect it. I'd have eight sheets of paper in front of me with basically the same paragraph on them. I was spending countless hours writing an essay, never feeling it was good enough, really struggling to finish. When I wasn't doing it I was worrying about it but I always felt I hadn't done enough. I was aiming for perfection. I'd delay and delay writing, and instead I'd read more and more in the hope that I would produce the perfect essay.

Eleanor's problems spread to other areas of her life.

> I felt like withdrawing. I wasn't at ease with people socially. Generally I didn't feel very good about myself. Talking in groups was very difficult. What I had to say didn't seem to be good enough. The course tutors expected participation in seminars and discussion and up until then I had felt fairly confident. But suddenly when I did speak I wasn't articulate and I wasn't clear. It was hard for me to start to talk and once I'd begun I'd lose confidence

halfway through what I was saying and dry up. It felt like I was on a downward spiral and I had no control as I fell.

Eleanor knows now some of the reasons for her change in mood. The ways she'd been taught to think academically at school were very different from the ways being put forward at college. She saw her method of thinking as being challenged. She also knew she'd been very successful at school – one of the brightest in the year. At college she was just one of many who were very bright.

A lot of my self-esteem was based on being academically successful to an unhealthy level. I felt as long as my work was OK I was OK. But fundamentally I didn't feel OK and when I went from being a star to being just one of many clever people, just average really, I couldn't cope.

I went home for Christmas and I was already in two minds about whether I could continue. I tried to talk with my parents about the possibility of taking a year off but they were completely panicked by the idea. They said, 'You can't possibly do that.' They were very frightened of anything out of the ordinary – and of me being vulnerable. They were just desperately saying, 'Keep going, keep going,' rather than helping me look at the different options I had.

That was a turning point for me. It was clear they couldn't support me as I struggled and I began to think I needed help from somewhere else. I went back and it was in the next term I had the worst moment. I had to go to a seminar with ten people in it. The tutor was a very aggressive man and he'd told us at the beginning that he expected us all to participate – he didn't want any 'shrinking violets' in his group. But I couldn't open my mouth. I was terrified and thinking, 'I can't stand being in this room. I've got to get out.' It was real panic. I was just praying for the hour to end. I was feeling sick and very frightened. My heart was racing, my mind was everywhere.

As soon as it ended I ran out of the room and into the women's toilets and burst into tears. I sat on the loo crying and worrying about what other people would think. The stress of internal conflict filled me. Part of me was saying, 'I don't want to be here, I don't want to be anywhere near this place,' while another part was saying, 'You have to be here. You can't leave.'

Throughout this time I was very tired. I wanted to be in bed all the time, cuddling myself with the covers pulled right over me. I had no energy, my limbs were heavy. In the end I couldn't stand the pressure of the inner conflict any more. I had to jump one way or the other and the only way was out. I felt that if I didn't have a break from the stress I'd probably do something to myself.

Luckily Eleanor knew of several other students who had been to see student counsellors attached to the college and she decided to go too. She thought this might give her the support she needed to go through with her decision.

More than anything else, the counsellor listened to me. She didn't tell me what to do although she did tell me the impressions she had of me and how she experienced me. The atmosphere was gentle and I remember at first just going there to cry.

By this time I could cope with the other students even less than I could before. I'd be walking through the college with my head down hoping no one would come up to me and say hello. I didn't want contact with anyone because I felt I'd have to perform and pretend I was OK and that would be a huge strain. I certainly wasn't able to let people know what was going on. I hated myself for feeling so bad – and I thought I was the only one who couldn't cope.

With the counsellor's help I focused my mind on the decision I had to make and I made it. She helped me put the wheels in motion to apply to take a year off. As soon as I'd made the decision I started to feel less stressed – I had some control back, I'd begun to take charge of the situation. Before I'd felt so vulnerable that if anyone had said a nasty word I thought I'd collapse. Now I started to feel much more positive.

Eleanor felt the counselling had been very useful but she also felt it wasn't going far enough for her. 'I wanted more than to be listened to, accepted and told I was OK. I wanted to explore the roots of my poor self-esteem more and she wasn't offering that.' She also had an experience with her counsellor which she found difficult to cope with. 'I went to see her one day and I could sense there was something wrong with her. I asked her if she was all right and she burst into tears about something that was happening in her life. That knocked my confidence in her. I didn't feel badly towards her but I knew I needed more.'

Eleanor then contacted a psychotherapist at a local health centre.

He helped me explore my relationship with my mum and the reasons why I felt so badly about myself. I could feel my self-confidence grow, although sometimes it was a difficult and painful process. It also helped me understand my mum more and helped me not to expect more from her than she could give me.

Eleanor took the year off and established a life for herself away from the college.

I got a job, enjoyed working and made a lot of close

friends. Academic success was no longer everything – and ironically that made it easier for me to return to college, to write essays more confidently and get a good degree.

For me, both counsellors were very useful. The first was supportive and helped me to get things that were terrifying me into perspective, and to make an important decision and see it through. As I began to feel better about myself I felt I wanted to know more about why this crisis was happening and why I felt so bad and I found another method of counselling to help me do that. I wonder now why I felt I had to struggle alone for so long.

ALTERNATIVE OR COMPLEMENTARY MEDICINE

Acupuncture

This traditional Chinese medicine can be used very successfully to treat conditions caused by stress and to promote calm. It works on the theory that Chi – or vital energy – flows in our bodies, concentrated in our meridians or vertical paths. Chi and blood move along the meridians carrying nourishment and strength. All organs and tissues have access to the meridians and both emotional and physical factors can restrict the flow, affecting our energy levels and our well-being.

Because the meridian system unifies all the parts of the body it is essential for the maintenance of harmonious balance. Chinese medicine isn't based on treating symptoms. Rather, it is based on the principle of reharmonising any bodily imbalance. A person who is well or 'in harmony' has no distressing symptoms and experiences mental and physical balance. When that person is ill the symptoms are only one part of a complete bodily imbalance that can be seen in other aspects of his or her life or behaviour.

Acupuncturists treat stress in its emotional and physical aspects. Classical theory recognises about 365 acupuncture points on the surface meridians of the body, each one having a defined therapeutic action. The practitioner chooses to work on those points that are most appropriate for treating a particular individual, and a typical treatment involves the insertion of around five to fifteen needles. Many are put off acupuncture because of the needles but they're of hair-like thinness and produce relatively little pain, sometimes none at all. The needles are made of stainless steel and are usually disposable.

Different emotions are linked to different organs of the body: the liver is linked to anger, the spleen to over-contemplation and worry, the kidney to fear, the heart to joy and over-excitement, and the lungs to grief. When any one state dominates over our internal experience or our outward behaviour this interferes with the conduct of our daily life and disrupts the smooth flow of Chi. The practitioner works to alter this.

If you're suffering from stress an acupuncturist may also give dietary advice as appropriate, recommend changes to your lifestyle or prescribe a combination of traditional Chinese herbs as part of a holistic programme.

The theory of acupuncture is obviously a long way from what most of us in the West are used to but many people swear by it.

Relaxation and Meditation

If you are able to give yourself time and allow yourself to slow down and feel the benefits, these are effective treatments for stress and anxiety. They involve changing the direction of the flow of attention. Most of the time attention is directed outwardly – putting us in touch with different forms of stress. But if, through relaxation or meditation, we direct our attention inwardly we disconnect from those external stresses. The body self-heals, relaxation responses take over and we feel at peace with ourselves.

One method of achieving this control over our responses is autogenic training – a Western rediscovery of some of the basic principles of Eastern meditation in which the participant learns to switch off the 'fight or flight' response to stress. Autogenics can be learnt in a class or from books or videos.

Mary

Mary, a young mother, feels autogenic training has helped her through some stressful times. For many years she had felt very stressed. She was overworking and was allowing her health to suffer with problems she felt were stress related, including colitis – inflammation of the colon – and shingles.

> Sometimes I worked from nine in the morning till eleven at night. I did a full-time job in an office with extra bar work in the evenings. My body was giving me warning signs that I was really stressing it out but I just carried on. I never felt I could take time off work or could lift my head up from it.

Mary was very close to her mother, who had recently died from cancer.

> Instead of sitting back and thinking about it I just kept ploughing on. There was a bit of my mother's death I hadn't dealt with – the impact of her absence on me – but I was too frightened to face this. Instead, I just put one foot in front of the other. I just kept moving. It was like being on a rollercoaster.
> My husband and I have a good relationship but when I tried to talk to him about how I was feeling it just ended up with me moaning rather than anything positive coming out. I said I wasn't happy but I never managed to sort anything out. I'd get into a real state and he'd be very calm and patient

and would walk round the park with me saying, 'Calm down,' but it needed to come from me. I needed to find a calmness in myself. And I couldn't.

In the end it was her body which cried for help and persuaded Mary to seek it.

When my mother was dying my colitis was bad and when she actually died it was terrible. I didn't know whether I was coming or going. I'd been from hospital department to hospital department and they all did tests. Something inside me was shouting out, 'Look what's happening in my life. Ask me what's happening in my life,' but nobody did.

Then I got pregnant. I was delighted to be expecting a baby but I also came to a big crisis. I knew something quite radical had to change in my life if I was going to have a child. I had been to see a homoeopathic doctor about my physical health and I would go and see her and cry. She said to me, 'You don't need treatment, you need to talk.' So for an hour a week I went to her and just talked to her. She said I had acute problems but they were emotional, not medical. She also mentioned she was involved with something called autogenics, which was a kind of self-based therapy. She said she didn't think I was ready to try it so soon after my mother died, but she felt if I went home and licked my wounds and allowed myself to heal, I'd be able to have a go when I felt better.

When Mary had worked through some of her grief for her mother she went back to train in autogenics.

My biggest feeling about it was, 'This won't work for me,' but in fact I relaxed in a way I've never relaxed before. It felt like a kind of self-hypnosis. We were taught to focus our minds into our bodies so that we were in a passive state. It sounds weird, I know, but it really worked. You tell yourself, 'My right arm is heavy.' Then you concentrate on what's happening in your right arm and by about week three it does feel heavy and you do that with various parts of the body. It's all about your mind going on to the backburner and focusing on where your body's at.

You start off by concentrating on every little bit of your body, relaxing the whole of you. Then you concentrate on individual parts of the body and have a routine each week taking on a few more parts. You have to practise the exercises three times a day at least. While you're doing this your mind throws up images which keep coming back. Mine almost made me feel sick – it was a shin and a foot and I had no idea what it meant. Then one day I was wearing a pair of sandals that my mother used to wear and I realised my image was of my mother's foot and leg. I also realised this was the first place her cancer was visible because her legs were very discoloured, which had been very disturbing to see. I felt it was obviously tied up with grieving for my mother – it was such a powerful image of her illness. Then once I'd realised what the image was about, it went away. I felt much calmer.

With autogenics we also learned to say affirmations to ourselves – 'I know I can heal myself,' is one. 'I love and accept my body completely' – I find it hard to say that one. 'I accept all my feelings as part of myself' – I find that easy to say but not so easy to believe in.

The system helped Mary find a calmness inside herself she hadn't felt before. This was soon put to the test when she faced a high-stress situation during the birth of her baby.

They induced me at ten and I went into labour at one in the morning. But they wouldn't let my husband Frank come on to the ward as it was a general ward and they wouldn't let me move to the labour ward until I was more dilated. All my ante-natal preparation had been based on him being with me and I really wanted him with me. I had never envisaged being by myself.

I nearly panicked and then I remembered my autogenics which were really useful. I managed to forget what was happening in my tummy and all the pain of childbirth – and concentrate on my right arm! I didn't need any painkillers at all. That must be the mark of a really, really successful deep relaxation system.

Mary says she still finds herself getting very stressed.

I don't use autogenics enough. I don't use it for the stress life throws up ordinarily. I only use it when I get really stressed up. So I feel I have a key to controlling stress but I don't use it. I've just had another attack of shingles which is a signal for me that I'm worrying about everything and not giving myself time to relax. I think I need a refresher course to help me use it more in my everyday life.

Massage

Massage is one of the best known de-stressors. It helps create a feeling of calm and well-being through rubbing the body's soft tissue, its muscles and ligaments. This can be relaxing, or relaxing and invigorating, depending on the kind of massage you choose. A massage can cover your whole body, or just your neck, shoulders and head. You can see a professional massage practitioner or you can be massaged by a partner or friend. You can even massage parts of yourself.

Everyone knows that massage is generally a good relaxant but one of its most important benefits is often not noted. Practitioner Tom Cooper, who operates in north and east London, says, 'One of the most important aspects of massage is that it slows people down. As with a lot of therapies, you get an hour which is just your time. Most people spend their time thinking, "What's going to happen next?" rather than living in the moment. With massage it's, "What's happening right now?" which is much more relaxed.'

Tom practises holistic massage, a popular method involving slow movements which get away from the normal speediness of stress and help the recipient slow right down and become in touch with their body.

'With stress the body starts to become a bit of an appendage. When we get in touch more with our body we get a sense of being grounded instead of being concentrated in a little ball on the top of the neck,' he says.

Also the intimacy and touch can take the person being massaged back to babyhood. 'They can think, "Someone is willing to touch me, to give me that caring." Through massage past traumas can come through. Stress is a type of protection, with the shoulders up, shoulders forward as a way of protecting the chest. If all those areas are massaged to release tensions and release the emotions held in there, and the area becomes more physically relaxed, there are strong psychological implications. It also adds to your awareness: "Oh yes, I'm holding my shoulders up all the time – I can let that go. I'm not in a life-threatening situation."'

Tom says having a massage has a big effect on him. 'I breathe a lot easier. I always have a sense of being able to sigh and let go of the business that's going on in my mind and all the things I think I have to be doing. There's a release of the shoulders, the body sinking down a bit more into the table – and an increase in self-esteem because I'm thinking, "I deserve to have some time to myself and receive some nurturing."'

'If other business comes into my mind during a massage, I see what it is – say, a shopping list – and then let it go and come back to what's happening at the moment and sensing what the massage practitioner is doing at that time. As with meditation, I stay with my breathing and with the point of focus and with massage the point of focus is touch. If I fall asleep, that's fine. Aware of what's going on and relaxed at the same time, and it's a very gentle awareness in comparison to what we're all doing most of the time in a harsh environment. I try to bring some of that gentle awareness with me into my daily life.'

Another well-known form of massage is Swedish massage, which again relies more on stroking and stretching than on the pummelling and percussion hacking which is the stereotype. 'It's useful for dealing with stress, especially if the massage is being carried out at a time when you can't relax completely afterwards. It's a very good way of bringing energy and blood flow to the muscles and waking people up and energising them. With people who are very tense, a lot of the tiredness and tension comes out in the form of just needing to sleep. This is a good way of releasing the tension while still keeping a person alert.'

If you are worried about taking your clothes off for your massage, or about how many you will have to take off, you can talk your questions and fears through with your practitioner. With another form of massage, Shiatsu, which involves massaging and pressuring the same meridian lines used in acupuncture, you can keep loose clothing on during the massage.

David

At his new job as an executive at a radio station, David felt his work had overtaken his life. Nothing was further from his mind than allowing himself an hour for a massage.

> I felt so shattered when I got home I'd watch telly like a moron or I went straight to bed. I didn't feel able to do anything else. If I'd been able to make

myself go swimming I'd have felt better or if I could have thought of doing anything that was fun to do. But I couldn't think of anything which wasn't to do with preparing myself to face the next day.

If I'd said to my boss, 'I need to get away one day a week at five,' I'm pretty sure in retrospect that would have been possible. At the time it would have felt as if I was asking for a million-pound handout. It certainly never occurred to me to say, 'This job is stressing me out.' I was in a powerful position and it would have felt as if I was being weak or sissy. No, I felt I had to be there every minute of the day. The working hours were incredibly long anyway and for some reason I felt the need to make them longer.

I suppose it was partly because my boss was there all the hours God sent that I felt I should be there too. My boss was actually pretty hopeless – he was inexperienced and didn't know what he was doing. So life was so grim for everybody I felt a duty to see it through. I couldn't sack my own boss so I felt quite powerless. All I needed was to change my environment for a bit – maybe to have a long weekend away or a short holiday to convalesce – and my battery would have been immediately recharged, but it was unthinkable. I felt they needed me to be there at work all the time.

I just kept thinking, 'Things will get better.' It's a bit like driving somewhere with very little petrol left in the tank and thinking, 'If I go faster I'll get there before the petrol runs out.' It's nonsense, of course, but I was thinking that by persevering really hard the end would come quicker. I knew I had a chance of a new job in August – life would begin again then.

David realised he was energyless, snappy and uninspired. He didn't realise he was very stressed.

I don't think I called it stress. I did recognise I was having a difficult time at work but I think I identified it as tiredness. I must have felt it was better to admit to that. If I'd admitted I was stressed it would have been like saying I was failing at work and I couldn't cope. 'Stress' for me conjures up pictures of people having nervous breakdowns and of their bosses saying, 'You can't give him or her another job. It's all too much for them.'

Ever since I was a child I've always given myself the message that I must be able to cope. If one of my staff had told me they were unhappy at work I'd have been upset about that and would want to do what I could to help them. I'd be one hundred per cent sympathetic. But if someone had told me they were stressed I'd have thought, 'If you can't stand the heat get out of the kitchen.' And that's what I'd have thought about myself, too. I think most people in this line of work respond to stress. It's what gives them a kick. Helps them perform to the best of their abilities.

Unusually for David, he found he was suffering from headaches nearly all the time.

I went to my doctor and he told me to take a couple of days off work but I felt I couldn't. Looking back to the consultation, I feel critical that he didn't suggest any lifestyle changes or exercises or anything which I think I might have listened to coming from him. I wanted him to give me some advice I could follow. Instead he gave me some muscle relaxants.

As for my diet, I was eating badly – stodgy, comfort food, anything I thought would keep me going for a couple of hours. I picture myself then eating a great lump of something in front of the telly. Not going out. Losing touch with people.

Wandering down his high street one Saturday David spotted a health centre which offered massages. Completely on a whim he thought he'd have a go and made an appointment for the next Wednesday. This was going against the rest of his feelings and attitudes – that he should be able to cope by himself, that just by charging forwards he'd get through.

> By that point I was feeling so bad I was determined to keep the appointment, although it was in work time – but then any time would have been work time! I had been massaged before and quite often I've fallen asleep on the massage table instantly because I felt so relaxed and looked after. This is of course a long way away from the way I usually feel because I admit I tend not to look after myself.

David managed to escape from work on the Wednesday afternoon with an ease that surprised him.

> I think a lot of people convince themselves that they're indispensable and this was quite clear to me when the dissension I had expected to follow my request for time off didn't materialise! I went into the centre, was shown to a room, took my clothes off and lay down with a towel over me. Then the masseur came in and started to massage me.

He had no idea of what was to happen next.

> I started to cry, almost straightaway. As soon as he started to loosen me up it felt like a big weight was being taken away from me. Every night it felt like such a relief to be lying down – my feet and ankles were sore from standing up for so much of the day and the rest of me just wanted to collapse. Here I felt the same relief and more. It felt like someone was paying me attention and looking after me –

something I don't do to myself, instead I spend my time concentrating on other people.

I wasn't crying about anything in particular or even because I was unhappy. I was just crying with the relief of having this burden taken away. Having the blood pushed round my body a bit felt good, too. It really seemed to be brightening me up. I was hardly aware of the man who was massaging me. It didn't occur to me to be embarrassed that I was crying in front of him – although usually I wouldn't feel good about crying in front of someone else. He just wasn't important. I was the important one.

After his massage, David booked a series straightaway.

I was much more aware of the stress in different parts of my body and also of the amount of tension I was feeling and the sense of caring I felt because someone else was touching me. I had reached the stage where I wanted to be looked after.

Aromatherapy

This process uses essential oils removed from plants to treat the individual. Each oil has a different smell and a different effect with various healing properties. Aromatherapy can be very relaxing and good for treating stress and for building up resistance to stress. The best way to take in the oils is through massage, either from a professional or by yourself or a partner. The oils can also be inhaled by adding a few drops to a bowl of hot water. Sometimes they can be taken internally – but very diluted in a tea or mixed in with herbs and spices. It is dangerous to take them undiluted by mouth. Adding them to your bath and soaking for at least ten minutes is also recommended.

The most effective essential oils for stress and stress-related symptoms according to expert Danièle Ryman in her excellent book *The Aromatherapy Handbook* (published by the C.W. Daniel Company) are:

- For anxiety – basil and marjoram.
- To help concentration – basil, bergamot, carnation, coriander, rosemary.
- For depression – angelica, basil, carrot, coriander, eucalyptus, ginger, lavender, mandarin, marjoram, mint, neroli and parsley.
- For insomnia – basil, camomile, lavender, mandarin, melissa, neroli, orange, rose, rosemary and thyme.
- To stop nightmares – basil, lemon, fennel, mint and rosemary.
- To shift a lack of interest in sex – aphrodisiac qualities in cinnamon, savory, ylang ylang, ginger, rose and sage.
- To prime the body for exercise, aid perspiration and encourage deep breathing – rosemary, ylang ylang, eucalyptus and benzoin.

Some aromatherapy oils should not be used if you are pregnant or suffer from epilepsy or other conditions.

Health Farms

These are no longer the puritan, sterile locations that the old stereotype suggests but more like places of pampering. Time spent at a health farm can do much to reduce stress levels and shake off dull routines. They are still not cheap – a stay in one is often seen as a replacement for rather than an addition to a holiday. In fact, a health farm could be more beneficial than a vacation. If holidays mean too much sun, rich food and too much drink, lost passports, airport delays and a foreign setting, a stay in a health farm will remove the stressful environment rather than replacing it with another one.

Victoria Barclay of the Inglewood Health Hydro in Kintbury, Berkshire, says, 'A health farm detoxifies the body through a variety of ways and so unconscious stress is released. The stressful environment of home or office is removed and so more conscious stress is released. We have very few people walking through the doors who aren't pretty uptight – a lot of bookings are only made two or three weeks before they arrive. Everyone coming to relax in the strict sense of the word – dressing gowns, make-up scraped off you, nothing to hide behind. To put on make-up and a posh track suit is almost out of place. The emphasis really is to be yourself.'

Inglewood provides four treatments a day including massage, a G5 mechanical massage, water treatments and heat treatments. Osteopathy, physiotherapy, a dietician, health and fitness experts, nurses and a doctor are also available. So are beauty treatments which help raise self-esteem. Food is healthy and plentiful. Alcohol is limited, apart from wine at the weekend, and smoking is discouraged.

'Some come after suffering bereavements, divorces, redundancies, or too much stress at work. By the time they leave they see things differently. To us the optimum is one week,' says Victoria Barclay. 'It's very relaxing to concentrate on yourself. Most people don't get the opportunity to focus entirely on their own needs – women especially consider this a selfish way to carry on.'

Yoga

This ancient method of keeping fit and relaxing helps to release physical and mental tension, thereby liberating energy. It's a good way to keep fit and yet it's not exhausting and has no age limit.

Yoga heightens awareness of each part of the body as you stretch as far as you can without risking injury. Then you stop and relax before going on to the next part of the body. All the while the body has time to recover and unwind. Yoga is also good for stress because it's non-competitive – it's about yourself and a personal sense of achievement.

It also calms the mind as well as the body. As you concentrate on what's happening to your body, you have less stress and fewer jumbled thoughts filling your mind.

You can reach a state of meditation during the routine, purely through concentrated thought.

Alexander Technique

Another popular alternative therapy excellent for stress, this technique corrects bad posture and brings the body back into alignment. The theory is that stress affects nerves, muscles, joints and bones so it's not enough just to concentrate on de-stressing the mind. Through the Alexander Technique, we change our reactions to everyday life, unlearning bad habits we've picked up in the way we stand, walk and sit. Working on the body is said to help the mind too, in that if you can correct a physical imbalance you can also correct mental stress which causes anxieties. A cycle is broken which began because it was stress and fear which initially made people adopt bad posture.

Other Therapies

OSTEOPATHY This technique uses manipulation and massage to help joints and muscles work smoothly and to de-stress them. As with the Alexander Technique, osteopaths believe that as posture improves, the state of mind improves.

REFLEXOLOGY A therapy based on the principle that stiffness or pain in particular zones of the feet and hands affect particular areas of the body. If there's stress in those parts of the body, reflexology can provide relief.

TRICHOLOGY Scalp disorders including patches of hair loss can be related to stress. A trichologist will treat and massage the scalp.

HERBALISM These remedies draw greatly on age-old techniques but are becoming very fashionable again. At the beginning of the century most drugs were based on herbs. Their retained popularity is partly because they are non-addictive, have no side-effects if used correctly and can have very impressive results. They can be helpful in treating nervous tension, depression, insomnia, stress and tension due to menstruation, nervous headaches and migraines. However, some may not be used during menstruation and some not used during pregnancy.

Herbs are usually taken in the form of an infusion (hot or boiling water is poured over them), a decoction (made by simmering herbs in water and then straining the solids away) or a tincture (made by soaking the herb in a mixture of alcohol and water, and taken diluted). Herbs can be bought from many health shops and from herbal suppliers but I would recommend you see a medical herbalist or buy a book about herbal remedies to find out details of which herbs might be relevant for you and how to prepare them.

HOMOEOPATHY The theory behind homoeopathy is that a substance poisonous in large quantities can cure in very small ones. The substance is taken in the form of pills, capsules, sachets of powders, sachets of granules, or liquids. Homoeopathic remedies can be bought ready prepared at health stores or a practitioner will give an individual diagnosis.

Peppermint and coffee should not be imbibed while you are taking a homoeopathic remedy. Leave a ten-minute gap before and after eating and drinking. For everyday ailments use the 6th potency (this will be marked on the packet). If your condition feels more serious, consult a practitioner.

If you're looking at buying homoeopathic remedies without the help of a practitioner I'd strongly recommend you also buy the booklet *Homoeopathy for the Family*, which may be found in the homoeopathy section of your health store and which gives an in-depth guide to medicines, which to take and how to take them.

USEFUL ADDRESSES

UK

Al-Anon/Alateen, 61 Great Dover Street, London SE1. Tel: 071 403 0888
Help for the families of problem drinkers.

Alcoholics Anonymous, General Service Office, PO Box 1, Stonebow House, York. Tel: 0904 644026
(London Region Tel: 071 352 3001)

Association of Sexual and Marital Therapists, PO Box 62, Sheffield SI0 3TS
Send an SAE for a list of therapists.

British Association for Counselling, 1 Regent Place, Rugby CV21 2PJ. Tel: 0788 578328
Provide details of counsellors near you, their specialised areas of work and their fees (if any).

British Migraine Association, 178a High Road, Byfleet, Weybridge, Surrey. Tel: 0932 52468

Council for Involuntary Tranquilliser Addiction (CITA), Cavendish House, Brighton Road, Waterloo, Liverpool L22 5NG. Tel: 051 525 2777
Helps those addicted to tranquillisers.

Cruse, 126 Sheen Road, Richmond, Surrey TW9 1UR. Tel: 081 940 4848
For bereavement counselling and care.

Eating Disorders Association, Sackville Place, 44 Magdalen Street, Norwich, Norfolk NR3 1 JE

Lifestyle Management, 13 Merton Hall Road, London SW19 3PP. Tel: 081 543 2086
Has produced Stress Sensors to measure your stress level, a Stress Release Audio Tape to help you learn to relax, and other useful items.

The Maisner Centre for Eating Disorders, PO Box 464, Hove BN3 2NB. Tel: 0273 729818/29334
Has produced a tape which offers help in stress release and beating compulsive eating.

Migraine Trust, 45 Great Ormond Street, London WC1N 3HZ. Tel: 071 278 2676

MIND, The National Association for Mental Health, 22 Harley Street, London W1N 2ED. Tel: 071 637 0741
Gives information over the phone, including referral to one of their 240 local groups, which may provide counselling, housing, drop-in centres or other facilities.

National Association for Pre-Menstrual Syndrome, 33 Pilgrims Way West, Otford, Sevenoaks, Kent. Tel: 0732 459378
Information Line Tel: 0227 763133

Parentline, Westbury House, 57 Hart Road, Thundersley, Essex SS7 3PD. Tel: 0268 757077
Helps parents under stress with their telephone helpline.

Parents Anonymous (London), 6 Manor Gardens, London N7 6LA. Tel: 071 263 8918
Lifeline for distressed parents.

Parent Network, 44 Caversham Road, London NW5 2DS. Tel: 071 485 8535
Organises support groups to help with parenting.

PAX (incorporating the Agoraphobia Information Service), 4 Manorbrook, London SE3 9AW. Tel: 081 318 5026.
Provides information about agoraphobia and general anxiety states, establishes contacts between self-help organisations and individual sufferers. Produces a newsletter.

Phobic Action, Claybury Grounds, Manor Road, Woodford Green, Essex 1G8 8PR. Tel: 0452 865021 or 081 559 2459

Relate (Marriage Guidance), Herbert Gray College, Little Church Street, Rugby, Warwickshire CV21 3AP. Tel: 0788 573241
Counselling help (you don't need to be married).

Relaxation for Living, 29 Burwood Park Road, Walton-on-Thames, Surrey KT12 5LH
Runs relaxation classes, correspondence courses on relaxation, has leaflets, books and tapes.

Spectrum, 7 Endymion Road, London N4 1EE. Tel: 081 341 2277/340 0426
Centre for humanistic psychotherapy.

Stress in Perspective, PO Box 359, London SW19 4XZ
Offers help in the workplace.

The Thanet Phobic Group, 47 Orchard Road, Westbrook, Margate, Kent CT9 5JS. Tel: 0843 33720
Countrywide support group with a monthly magazine.

Unwind, Melrose, 3 Alderlea Close, Gilesgate, Durham DH1 1DS. Tel: 091 384 2056
Helps phobic people and those suffering from stress.

Westminster Pastoral Foundation, 23 Kensington Square, London W8 5HN. Tel: 071 937 6956
Provides counselling.

Women's Therapy Centre, 6 Manor Gardens, London N7 6LA. Tel: 071 263 6200.

ALTERNATIVE AND COMPLEMENTARY MEDICINE

Association of Reflexologists, 110 John Silkin Lane, London SE8 5BE
A register of practitioners' costs.

British Acupuncture Association, 34 Alderney Street, London SW1 4EU. Tel: 071 834 1012 or 834 6229
Will send a register of their members.

British Association for Autogenic Training, 101 Harley Street, London W1. Tel: 071 935 1811

British Complementary Medicine Association, St Charles Hospital, Exmoor Street, London W10 6DZ. Tel: 081 964 1205

British Homoeopathic Association, 27a Devonshire Street, London W1N 1RJ. Tel: 071 935 2163

British Wheel of Yoga, 1 Hamilton Place, Boston Road, Sleaford, Lincs NG34 7ES. Tel: 0529 306851

Council for Complementary and Alternative Medicine, 179 Gloucester Place, London NW1 6DX. Tel: 071 724 9103

General Council and Register of Consultant Herbalists, Grosvenor House, 40 Seaway, Middleton-on-Sea, West Sussex PO22 7SA. Tel: 0243 586012

General Council and Register of Osteopaths, 56 London Street, Reading, Berks RG1 4SQ. Tel: 0734 576585

Institute of Complementary Medicine, PO Box 194, London SE16 1QZ. Tel: 071 237 5165

National Institute of Medical Herbalists, 9 Palace Gate, Exeter, Devon EX1 1JA. Tel: 0392 426022

Nationwide Institute of Psychosexual Medicine, 11 Chandos Street, Cavendish Square, London W1M 9DE. Tel: 071 580 0631
Will help you find an accredited sex therapist.

Natural Therapeutic and Osteopathic Society, 14 Marford Road, Wheathampstead, Herts AL4 8AS. Tel: 0582 833950

Redwood Women's Training Association, 5 Spennithorne Road, Skellow, Doncaster, South Yorkshire DN6 8PF. Tel: 0302 337151
Runs assertiveness training classes.

Society of Homoeopaths, 2 Artizan Road, Northampton NN1 4HU. Tel: 0604 21400

Society of Teachers of the Alexander Technique, 20 London House, 266 Fulham Road, London SW10 9EL. Tel: 071 351 0828

Please send a stamped addressed envelope when writing to any of the above organisations.

CANADA

Acupuncture Foundation of Canada, 5 Roughfield Cr, Toronto ON M1S 4K3. Tel: (416) 291 4317

Alcohol and Drug Concerns Inc, (also known as Concerns Canada), 11 Progress Avenue 200, Scarborough ON M1P 4S7. Tel: (416) 293 3400

Alcohol and Drug Dependency Information and Counselling Services (Manitoba), 2471 1/2 Portage Avenue, 2 Winnipeg MB R3J 0N6. Tel: (204) 831 1999

Canadian Centre for Stress and Wellbeing, 181 University Avenue, 1202 Toronto ON M5H 3M7. Tel: (416) 363 6204

Canadian Guidance and Counselling Association, 55 Parkdale Avenue, Ottawa ON K1Y 4G1. Tel: (613) 728 3281

Canadian Institute of Stress, 1235 Bay Street, Toronto ON M5R 3K4. Tel: (416) 961 8575
Parental Stress Services.

Canadian Osteopathic Aid Society, 575 Waterloo St, London ON N6B 2R2. Tel: (519) 439 5521

Canadian Society of Homoeopathy, 87 Meadowland Drive, WNepean ON K2G 2R9. Tel: (613) 723 1533

Canadian Society of Teachers of the FM Alexander Technique, 2181 Avenue Road, Toronto ON M5M 4B8. Tel: (416) 487 0567

Parents Anonymous, PO Box 843, Burlington ON L7R 3Y7. Tel: (416) 333 3971

Parents without Partners, PO Box 1218, Stn AOshawa ON L1J 5Z1. Tel: (416) 436 2255

Women's Counselling and Referral and Education Centre, 525 Bloor St W, Toronto ON M0M 0M0. Tel: (416) 534 7502

AUSTRALIA

Alcoholics Anonymous, 127 Edwin Street, Croydon, New South Wales 2132. Tel: (02) 799 1199A1

Alcohol and Drug Dependence Services, FreeCall, (008) 177 833-24-hour information and counselling.

Anon Family Groups, PO Box 1002H, Melbourne, Victoria 3001. Tel: (03) 650 3368/329 0105
Support for the families of alcoholics.

Australian Acupuncture Association, 275 Moggill Road, Indooroopilly, Queensland 4068. Tel: (07) 378 9377

Australian Institute of Homoeopathy, 21 Bulah Close, Berowra Heights, New South Wales 2082. Tel: (02) 456 3602

Australian Osteopathic Association, 4 Collins Street, Melbourne, Victoria. Tel: (03) 650 3736

Canberra Marriage Guidance Council, 15 Hall Street, Lyneham, Canberra 2602. Tel: (06) 257 3273

Dial-A-Mum of Australia, PO Box 241, Wahroonga, New South Wales 2067. Tel: (02) 477 6777
Voluntary association of mothers who offer a telephone counselling and guidance service.

Lifeline, 148 Lonsdale Street, Melbourne, Victoria 3000. Tel: (03) 662 1000
Crisis telephone counselling, information and referral service.

Marriage Guidance Council of New South Wales, 5 Sera Street, Lane Cove, New South Wales 2066. Tel: (02) 418 8800

Marriage Guidance Council of South Australia, 55 Hutt Street, Adelaide, South Australia 5000. Tel: (08) 223 4566

Marriage Guidance Council of Western Australia, PO Box 1289, West Perth, Western Australia 6872. Tel: (09) 321 5801

National Herbalists Association of Australia, PO Box 65, Kingsgrove, New South Wales 2208. Tel: (02) 502 2938

Northern Territory Marriage Guidance Council, PO Box 4193, Darwin, Northern Territory 0801. Tel: (089) 816676

Queensland Marriage Guidance Council, 159 St Pauls Terrace, Brisbane, Queensland 4000. Tel: (07) 831 2005

Tasmania Marriage Guidance Council, 306 Murray Street, Hobart, Tasmania 7000. Tel: (002) 313141

Victoria Marriage Guidance Council, 146 Princess Street, Kew, Victoria 3101. Tel: (03) 853 5354

INDEX